Geology Activity Book for Kids

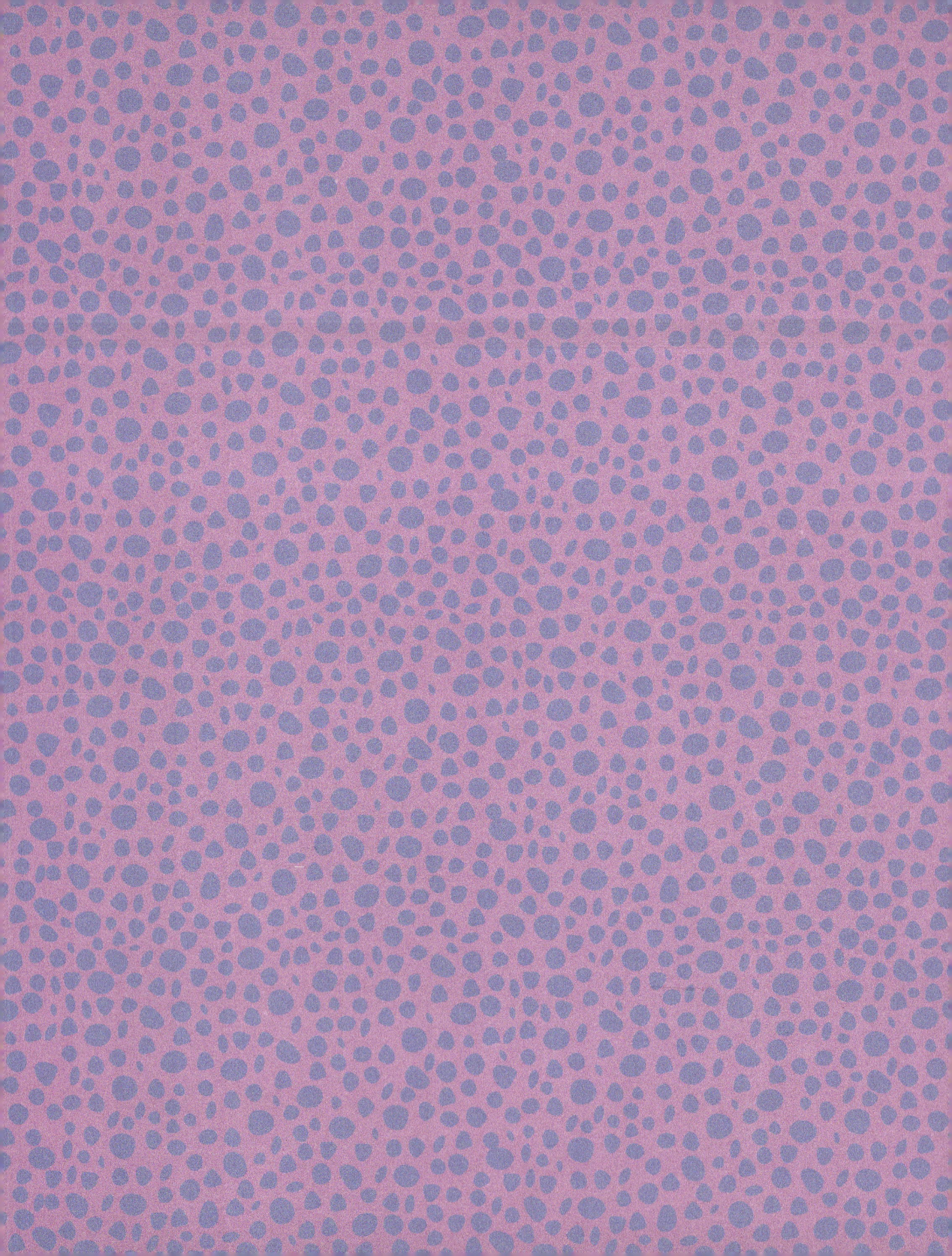

GEOLOGY ACTIVITY BOOK
for kids | Ages 5 to 7

Hands-On Fun Exploring Rocks, Minerals, and the Earth's Surface

MEGHAN VESTAL

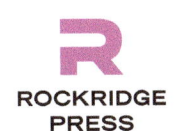

ROCKRIDGE PRESS

This book is dedicated to my daughter. I can't wait to explore this world with you!

Copyright © 2022 by Rockridge Press, Oakland, California

No part of this publication may be reproduced, stored in a retrieval system, or transmitted in any form or by any means, electronic, mechanical, photocopying, recording, scanning, or otherwise, except as permitted under Sections 107 or 108 of the 1976 United States Copyright Act, without the prior written permission of the Publisher. Requests to the Publisher for permission should be addressed to the Permissions Department, Rockridge Press, 1955 Broadway, Suite 400, Oakland, CA 94612.

Limit of Liability/Disclaimer of Warranty: The Publisher and the author make no representations or warranties with respect to the accuracy or completeness of the contents of this work and specifically disclaim all warranties, including without limitation warranties of fitness for a particular purpose. No warranty may be created or extended by sales or promotional materials. The advice and strategies contained herein may not be suitable for every situation. This work is sold with the understanding that the Publisher is not engaged in rendering medical, legal, or other professional advice or services. If professional assistance is required, the services of a competent professional person should be sought. Neither the Publisher nor the author shall be liable for damages arising herefrom. The fact that an individual, organization, or website is referred to in this work as a citation and/or potential source of further information does not mean that the author or the Publisher endorses the information the individual, organization, or website may provide or recommendations they/it may make. Further, readers should be aware that websites listed in this work may have changed or disappeared between when this work was written and when it is read.

For general information on our other products and services or to obtain technical support, please contact our Customer Care Department within the United States at (866) 744-2665, or outside the United States at (510) 253-0500.

Rockridge Press publishes its books in a variety of electronic and print formats. Some content that appears in print may not be available in electronic books, and vice versa.

TRADEMARKS: Rockridge Press and the Rockridge Press logo are trademarks or registered trademarks of Callisto Media Inc. and/or its affiliates, in the United States and other countries, and may not be used without written permission. All other trademarks are the property of their respective owners. Rockridge Press is not associated with any product or vendor mentioned in this book.

Interior and Cover Designer: Lisa Forde
Art Producers: Tom Hood and Sue Bischofberger
Editor: Maxine Marshall
Production Editor: Holland Baker
Production Manager: Riley Hoffman

Illustrations and activities © 2021 Collaborate Agency, except p. 4; © Bruce Rankin, p. 4.

Photography used under license from shutterstock.com, cover and pp. 7, 10, 31, 34 (except aquamarine), and 55; © Ted Kinsman/Science Source, pp. 1 and 16; used under license from iStockPhoto.com, pp. 13, 19, 22, 28, 46, and 52; © Reid Dalland/Alamy Stock Photo, p. 25; aquamarine on p. 34 used under license from 123RF; © Roberto Nistri/Alamy Stock Photo, p. 37; © PF-(usna)/Alamy Stock Photo, p. 40; © EyeEm/Alamy Stock Photo, p. 43; © The Protected Art Archive/Alamy Stock Photo, p. 49.

Author photo courtesy of Ben Vestal Video Production

Paperback ISBN: 978-1-63878-072-4
eBook ISBN: 978-1-63807-669-8
R0

Contents

DEAR PARENTS AND TEACHERS **vi**

All about Geology 1

Hard Core: The Structure of Earth **4**

Let's Rock: Types of Rocks **7**

Rock and Roll: The Rock Cycle **10**

All Mine: Minerals **13**

Glow in the Dark: Fluorescent Minerals **16**

Let's Rock at School: Geology in the Classroom **19**

Rock Around the House: Geology at Home **22**

Crystal Clear: Crystal Shapes and Structures **25**

What's Inside a Rock: Geodes **28**

Pretty Precious: Gems and Gemstones **31**

Happy Birthday: Birthstones **34**

Fantastic Planet: Fossils **37**

Shake It Up: Earthquakes **40**

Hot Lava: Volcanoes **43**

Peak to Peak: Mountains **46**

Water, Water Everywhere: Rivers, Streams, and Oceans **49**

Wet and Wild: Weathering **52**

Moving On: Erosion **55**

ANSWER KEY **59**
INDEX OF SKILLS **61**

Dear Parents and Teachers

Imagine taking your child on a journey to the center of the Earth or on an expedition to discover fossils. It's possible with this book!

I taught elementary school for several years before starting a curriculum company in 2015. Throughout my 15 years working in education, I have consistently seen the benefit of helping kids discover the world around them through hands-on exploration.

I hate to admit that when I started teaching, I was certain the "rock unit" would be the most boring of the school year. I couldn't have been more wrong. I discovered that geology is one of the best science units for hands-on learning. Kids are naturally curious about the Earth. They want to know what the Earth is made of and how it formed. Most kids also love going outside and getting dirty. Studying geology is the perfect way to blend learning with that natural desire to dig in the dirt.

Geology Activity Book for Kids was designed to empower kids to learn about the Earth through investigation. The book includes 19 sections, each tied to a central geology concept. Your child will discover topics like the layers of the Earth, rocks and minerals, fossils, landforms, and much more. Each section provides detailed information and fun facts with an emphasis on learning through doing. Experiments, puzzles, coloring activities, and other hands-on fun are incorporated into each section.

It is my sincere hope that this book will spark your child's interest in learning more about the world around them.

—Meghan Vestal

All about Geology

Have you ever looked at rocks or dug in the dirt? If so, you've been a geologist! Geology is the study of Planet Earth. We study the Earth to learn how it formed, what it is made of, and how it changes. Geology tells us about Earth's past and Earth's future.

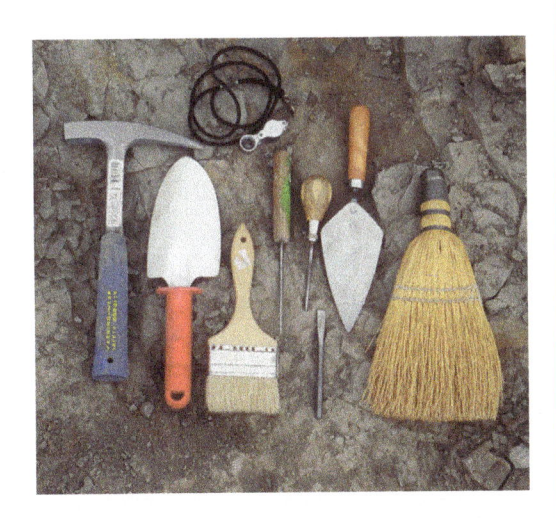

GEOLOGISTS' TOOLS HELP THEM DIG IN THE DIRT AND CAREFULLY REMOVE WHAT THEY FIND.

5 FUN FACTS

1. A person who studies geology is called a geologist.

2. Geology tells us what Earth looked like more than four billion years ago.

3. Geologists predict what Earth will look like in the future.

4. Geology affects every person. It controls how food is grown. It also affects our air and water.

5. Geologists use tools like brushes, shovels, notebooks, cameras, and bulldozers to study the Earth.

ACTIVITY

Use what you have learned about geology and geologists to complete the puzzle. Flip back to page 1 if you need help finding the answers.

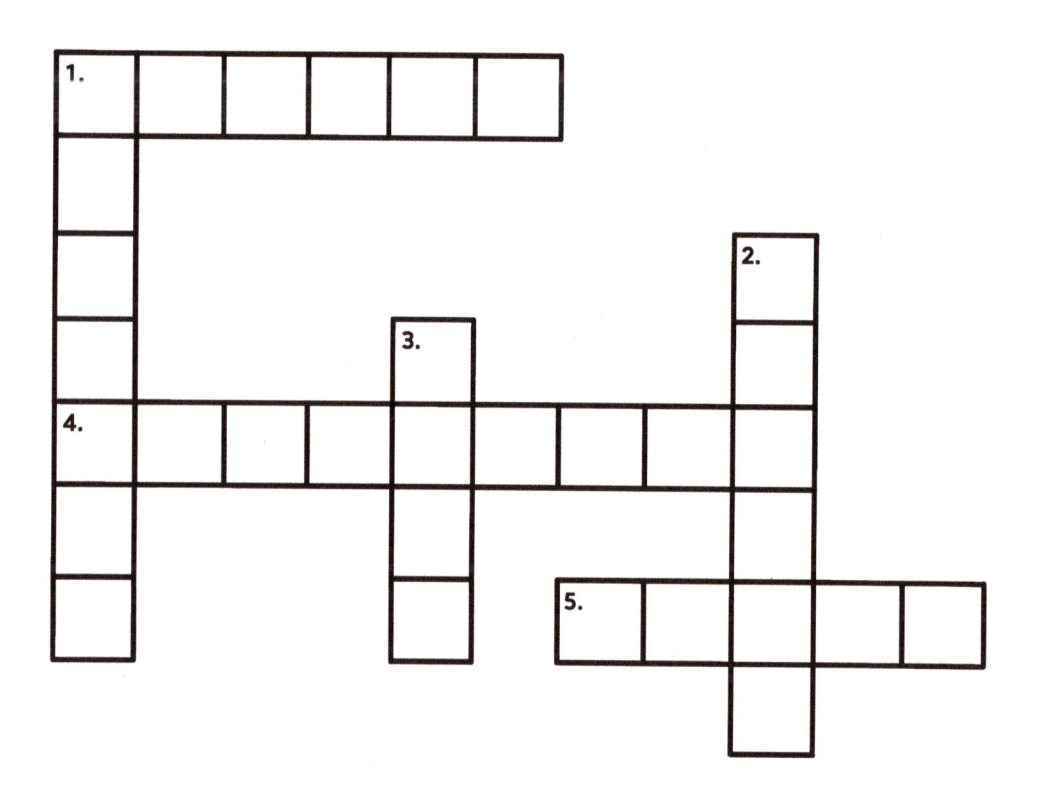

Across

1 A tool used by geologists to take pictures of rocks, minerals, and soil.

4 A person who studies geology.

5 Geology is the study of the _____.

Down

1 The Earth _____ over time.

2 Geology tells about Earth's past and _____.

3 The Earth is more than _____ billion years old.

GEOLOGY ACTIVITY BOOK FOR KIDS

GEOLOGY IN ACTION

Since geology is the study of the Earth, you can be a geologist anywhere that you can find rocks or **landforms**, like hills and rivers! Are there rocks near your home?

What you'll need:
Camera

What to do:

1. Ask an adult to join you on a walk outside.

2. Use the camera to take pictures of five things related to geology. This could include rocks, minerals, or landforms. You could also take pictures of places where the Earth has moved or changed.

3. Talk about what you see. How do you think these things formed? What could have caused the Earth to change?

4. Share your pictures with others.

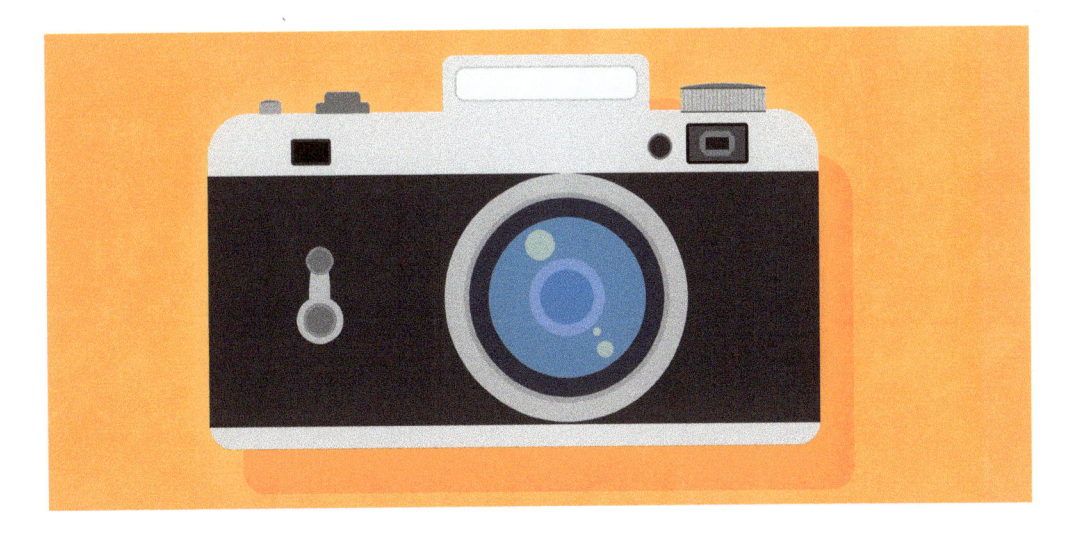

Hard Core:
The Structure of Earth

Imagine you could cut out a slice from **Planet Earth**, like a slice from an apple. What would you find? The Earth has four layers. Some layers are thick and some are thin. Each layer is made of different materials, and each layer affects the others. Changes deep inside the Earth create changes on the surface.

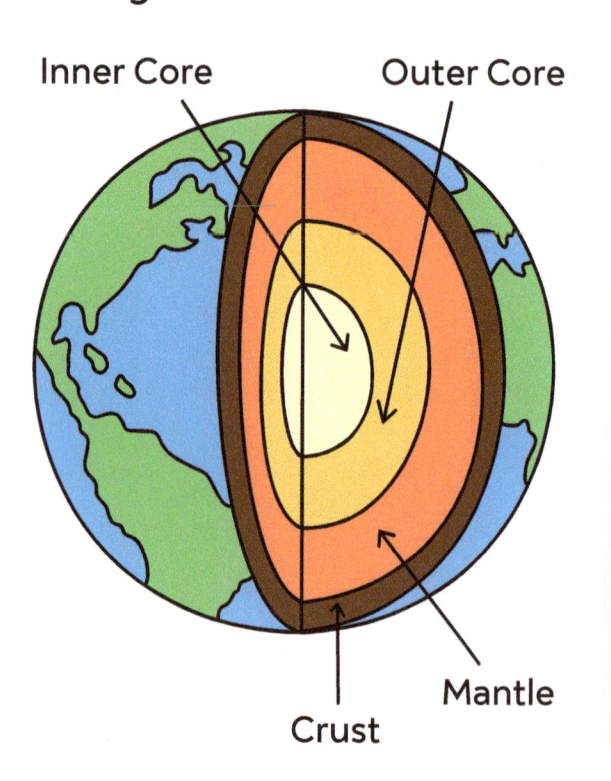

Inner Core   Outer Core

Crust   Mantle

5 FUN FACTS

1. The **inner core** is a ball of metal at the center of Earth. It is as hot as the Sun but doesn't melt.

2. The **outer core** is liquid and flows around the inner core.

3. The **mantle** is the biggest layer. It is made of both solid moving rocks and melted rock, called magma.

4. The **crust** is where we live. This top layer is thin, and more than half of it is under the oceans.

5. Since the core is so deep inside Earth, geologists study earthquakes to learn about it.

ACTIVITY

Draw a line to match each of Earth's layers to the correct descriptions.

Inner Core	Where you live
Outer Core	A ball of solid metal
Mantle	Liquid metal
Crust	The biggest layer

GEOLOGY IN ACTION

Geologists learn about the Earth by taking core samples. These samples show layers of rocks and soil. In this fun activity, you'll drill "core samples" from candy bars.

What you'll need:

Layered candy bar, like a SNICKERS or Milky Way

Paper plate

Clear plastic straw

Paper towel

What to do:

1. Unwrap the candy bar. Put it on the paper plate.

2. Poke the straw all the way through the candy bar from the top.

3. Gently pull out the straw from the candy bar.

4. Wipe off the outside of the straw with the paper towel.

5. Identify each layer of your core sample that is now inside the straw.

Let's Rock:
Types of Rocks

Not all rocks are made the same. There are three ways rocks are created. **Igneous** rocks are made when lava cools and hardens. **Sedimentary** rocks are made of tiny rocks, minerals, and even bits of ancient plants and animals all pressed together. **Metamorphic** rocks are made inside Earth when heat and pressure turn old rocks into new rocks.

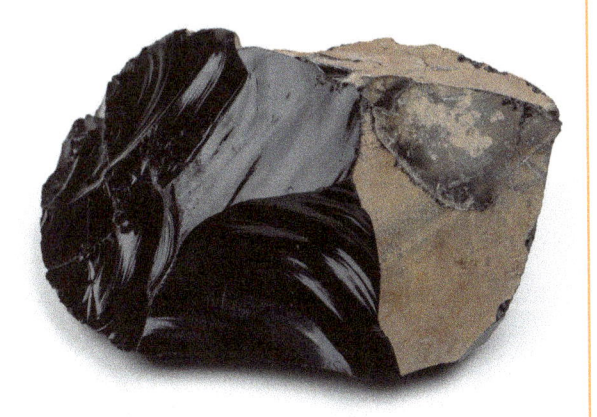

OBSIDIAN IS AN IGNEOUS ROCK THAT LOOKS LIKE SMOOTH, BLACK GLASS.

5 FUN FACTS

1. Lava still inside Earth is called magma. Igneous rocks are made both outside and inside of Earth.

2. Wind and water break rocks into pieces called **sediments**. Sedimentary rocks are made of lots of tiny sediments.

3. Sedimentary rocks often contain fossils. Fossils are what's left of plants and animals that lived long ago.

4. Metamorphic rocks can be made from igneous rocks, sedimentary rocks, or other metamorphic rocks.

5. Humans use rocks to make roads, electricity, tiles, and even toothpaste.

ACTIVITY

Read the description of each type of rock. Then color in the rock outline to match the description. You may want to look at rocks outside or on the internet for ideas.

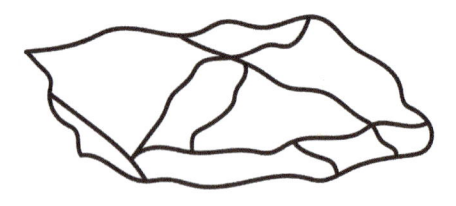

Igneous
Igneous rocks are dark colors. Most are smooth. Some look glassy. They may have small crystals or no crystals at all. Some igneous rocks have small holes all over.

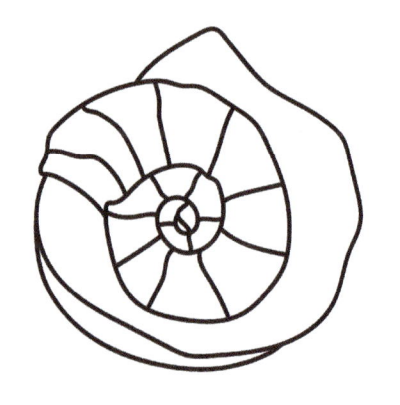

Sedimentary
Sedimentary rocks can be many different colors. They can be brown, yellow, white, red, or gray. You can usually see other rocks or sediments within them. Some sedimentary rocks have fossils in them.

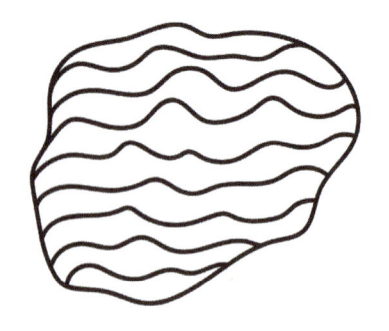

Metamorphic
Metamorphic rocks can be many different colors, such as black, gray, green, white, or red. You can usually see wavy lines in them. Most metamorphic rocks have crystals.

GEOLOGY IN ACTION

In this activity, you will use candy to model how sedimentary rocks form. Use your model to tell a friend about sedimentary rocks.

What you'll need:

3 Starburst candies (different colors)

What to do:

1. Unwrap the candies.

2. Hold the candies between your hands for several seconds. The heat from your hands will make them soft so that you can easily pull them apart.

3. Pull each candy apart into pieces, or "sediments." Each candy should break into three to four pieces.

4. Make a large ball or "rock" by sticking the pieces together. Can you see the different sediments?

Rock and Roll:
The Rock Cycle

Rocks change over time. Lava cools down and becomes igneous rocks. Wind and water break rocks into sediments that eventually make sedimentary rocks. Rocks get pushed deeper in the crust where heat and pressure change them to metamorphic rocks. Even deeper, they melt into magma, which erupts from volcanoes as lava to form igneous rocks again.

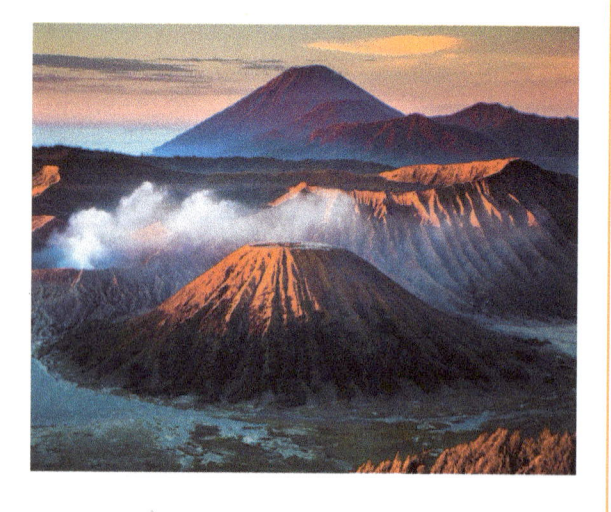

5 FUN FACTS

1. Rocks are always changing. An igneous rock wasn't always an igneous rock. It was a different rock in the past and will change again in the future.

2. It takes thousands or millions of years for rocks to change form.

3. The rock cycle does not always move in the same direction.

4. The rock cycle wouldn't exist without water. Water breaks down and moves rocks.

5. The rock cycle also wouldn't exist without magma. Magma forms and moves rocks.

ACTIVITY

Trace the lines to show the rock cycle. Do the lines always move in the same direction? Tell a friend how each of the rocks can change form.

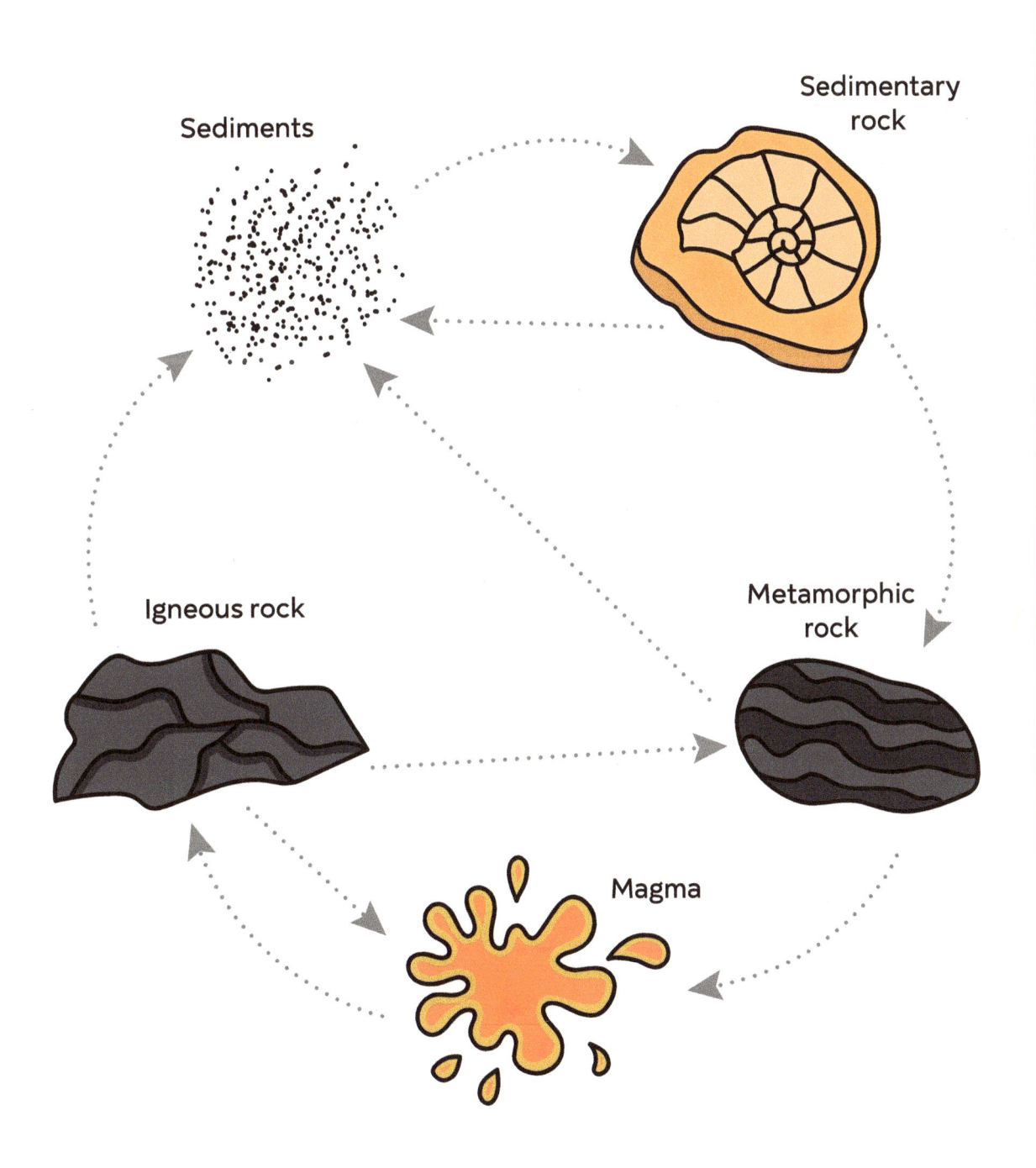

Sediments

Sedimentary rock

Igneous rock

Metamorphic rock

Magma

THE ROCK CYCLE 11

GEOLOGY IN ACTION

You will use crayons to model the rock cycle. Be sure to have an adult help with each step of this activity.

What you'll need:

3 crayons (different colors)

Cheese grater

Aluminum foil

Small frying pan

Stove

What to do:

1. Peel the paper labels off the crayons. Imagine the crayons are igneous rocks that are being broken down by wind and rain. Using the cheese grater, grate the "igneous rocks" over the aluminum foil.

2. Push the shavings into a pile. Place a piece of the foil on top. Using your hands, push down as hard as you can for one minute. Peel away the foil. You created a sedimentary rock.

3. Ask an adult to help you turn on the stove to medium heat. Set the pan on the stove. Place the foil with the "sedimentary rock" in the hot pan until it melts.

4. Turn off the stove. Watch the crayon cool. Now you've created a "metamorphic rock."

All Mine: Minerals

Rocks can be all kinds of colors! But no matter how different they look, all rocks are made of minerals. Minerals are solid objects that are not created by living things. We use minerals each day to cook, clean, and do schoolwork. What minerals can you find?

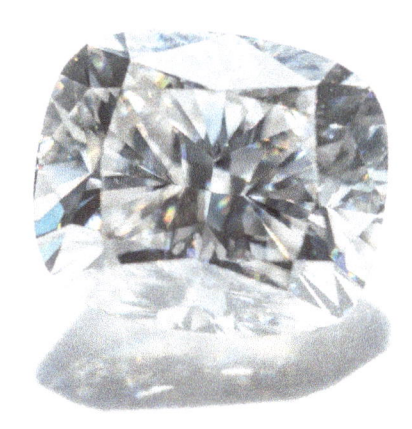

THE MINERAL DIAMOND IS VERY HARD. THE ONLY THING THAT CAN SCRATCH A DIAMOND IS ANOTHER DIAMOND.

5 FUN FACTS

1. There are more than four thousand kinds of minerals.

2. Each type of mineral is made in nature in a different way. Some are made inside Earth, and some are made on Earth's surface.

3. Jewelry is made of minerals. Diamonds, gold, silver, and quartz are all minerals.

4. Your home is made of minerals. Windows are made from quartz. Walls and cement are made from a mineral called calcite.

5. Sulfur is an explosive mineral. It is used to make fireworks.

ACTIVITY

A diamond is a beautiful mineral that people use to make jewelry. Diamonds can be found buried inside Earth or behind cave walls. Trace the maze to help the miner find the diamond.

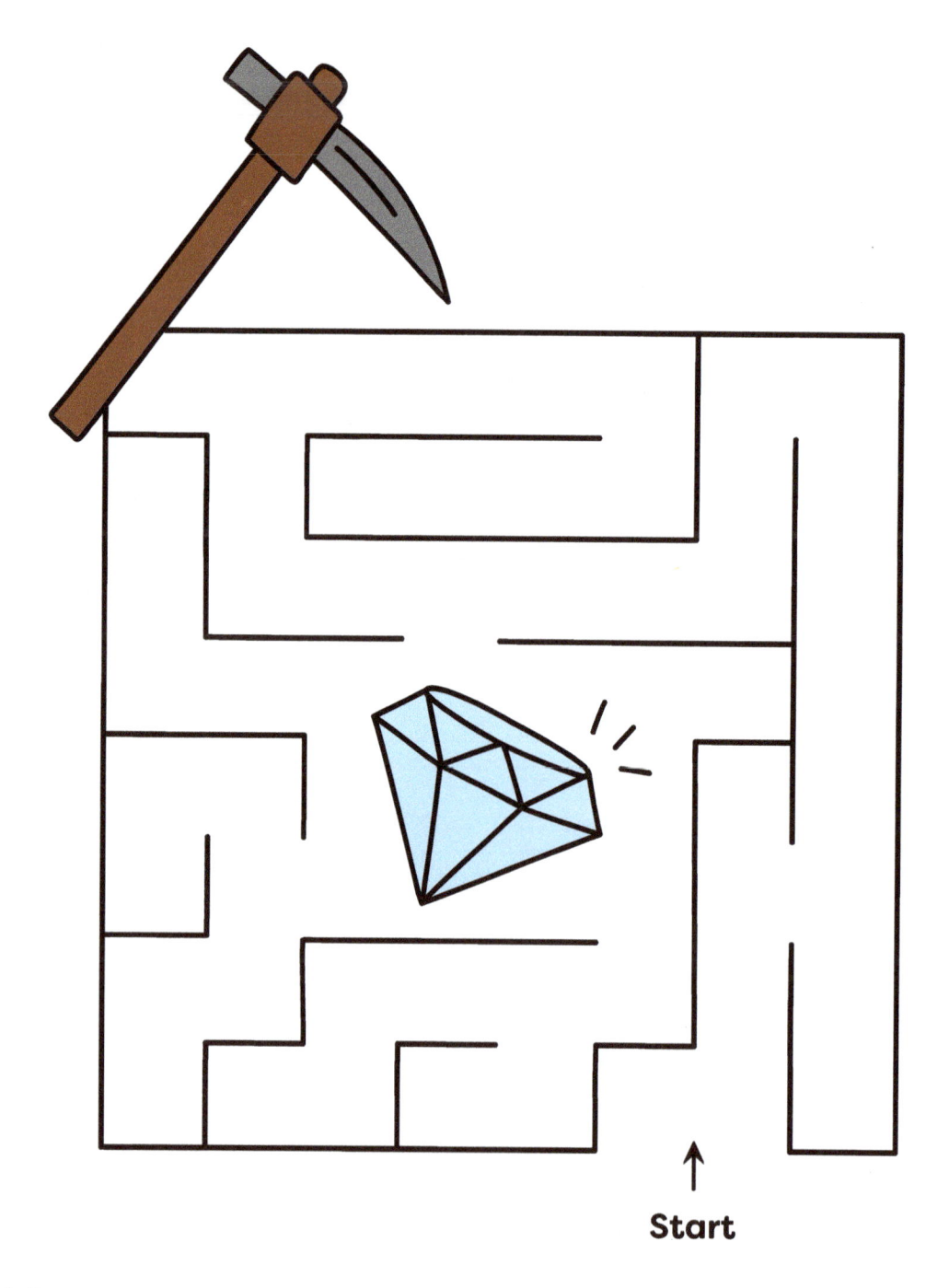

Start

GEOLOGY IN ACTION

Lots of minerals are found near water. Explore how geologists find minerals in rivers and lakes!

What you'll need:

Minerals, like quartz or mica (you can use quartz beads from your local craft store)

Medium-size plastic container

Sand or soil

Water

Fine-mesh strainer

What to do:

1. Scatter the minerals in the bottom of the container.

2. Cover the minerals with the sand or soil. Then fill the container halfway with the water.

3. Scoop the whole mixture into the mesh strainer. Slowly shake the strainer back and forth over the container, so that the sand and water drain out. How long does it take to find all the minerals?

Glow in the Dark:
Fluorescent Minerals

Minerals come in many shapes and colors, but some are also fluorescent. That means that if you hold one under an ultraviolet or black light, it will glow! Fluorescent minerals can glow green, purple, orange, blue, or red. They are beautiful and very rare.

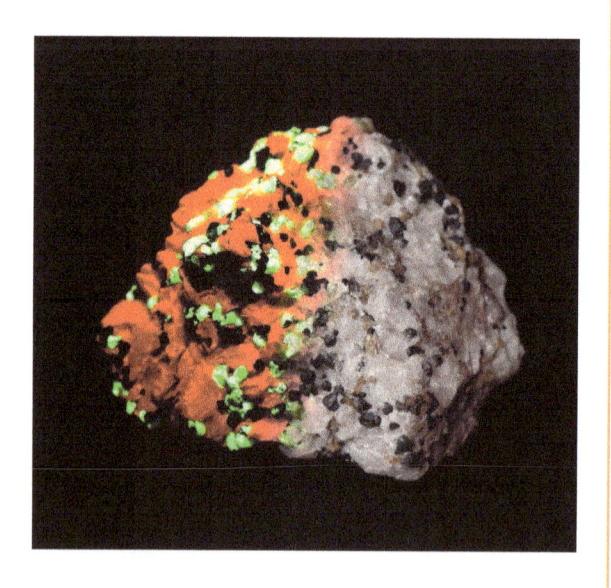

CALCITE IS A FLUORESCENT MINERAL THAT GLOWS RED OR GREEN.

5 FUN FACTS

1. Fluorescent minerals form when they touch certain other minerals or metals called **activators**.

2. Different activators cause fluorescent minerals to glow in different colors.

3. The term **fluorescent** comes from the mineral fluorite.

4. There are thousands of types of minerals but only about five hundred are fluorescent.

5. More fluorescent minerals have been discovered in New Jersey than anywhere else in the world.

ACTIVITY

A geologist discovers many minerals in a cave. When she holds them under an ultraviolet light, some glow and some do not. She arranges the minerals to form two patterns. Complete the patterns by coloring the next three minerals.

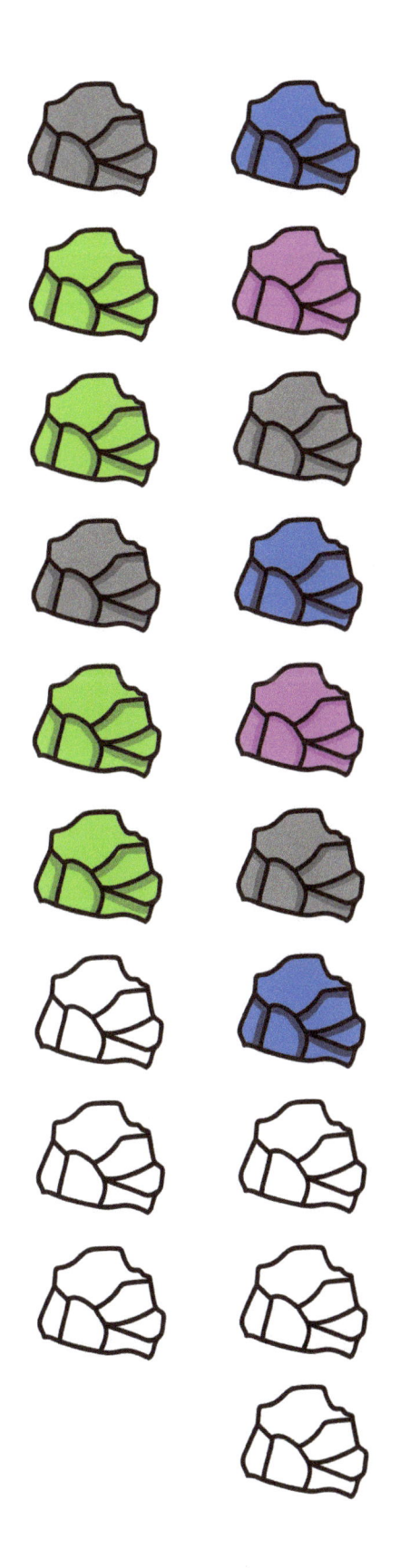

FLUORESCENT MINERALS **17**

GEOLOGY IN ACTION

You can make objects around your house glow just like fluorescent minerals!

What you'll need:

Clear jar, large enough for the egg

White vinegar

Highlighter pen

1 egg

Flashlight

What to do:

1. Fill the jar halfway with the vinegar.

2. Ask an adult to break the highlighter open and remove the ink pad. Squeeze the ink pad to get as much ink as possible into the jar.

3. Carefully place the egg in the jar. Leave it on the kitchen counter for three days.

4. When eggshell pieces start floating, remove the egg. Rinse away any remaining shell and dry.

5. Shine the flashlight on the egg in a dark room. Watch it glow!

Let's Rock at School:
Geology in the Classroom

Take a look around your classroom. You just looked at lots of different rocks and minerals! Blackboards are sometimes made from a rock called slate. The chalk used to write on it is made from a mineral called calcite. What other rocks and minerals do you see?

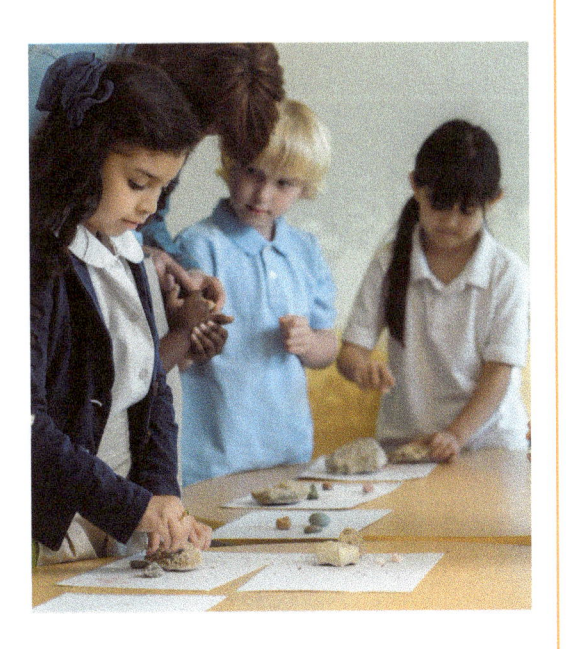

5 FUN FACTS

1. Pencil lead is made from a mineral called graphite.

2. More than 60 different minerals are used to build school computers.

3. Take a walk around the school. The hard floors are made from rocks, such as sandstone.

4. Stop in at the nurse's office. Rocks and minerals are there, too! Minerals, such as calcite, are used to make medicine.

5. Is your school made of bricks? Bricks are made from a rock called shale.

GEOLOGY IN THE CLASSROOM

ACTIVITY

All of these objects can be found in a classroom. Circle the objects that are made from rocks or minerals. Flip to page 19 if you need help finding the answers.

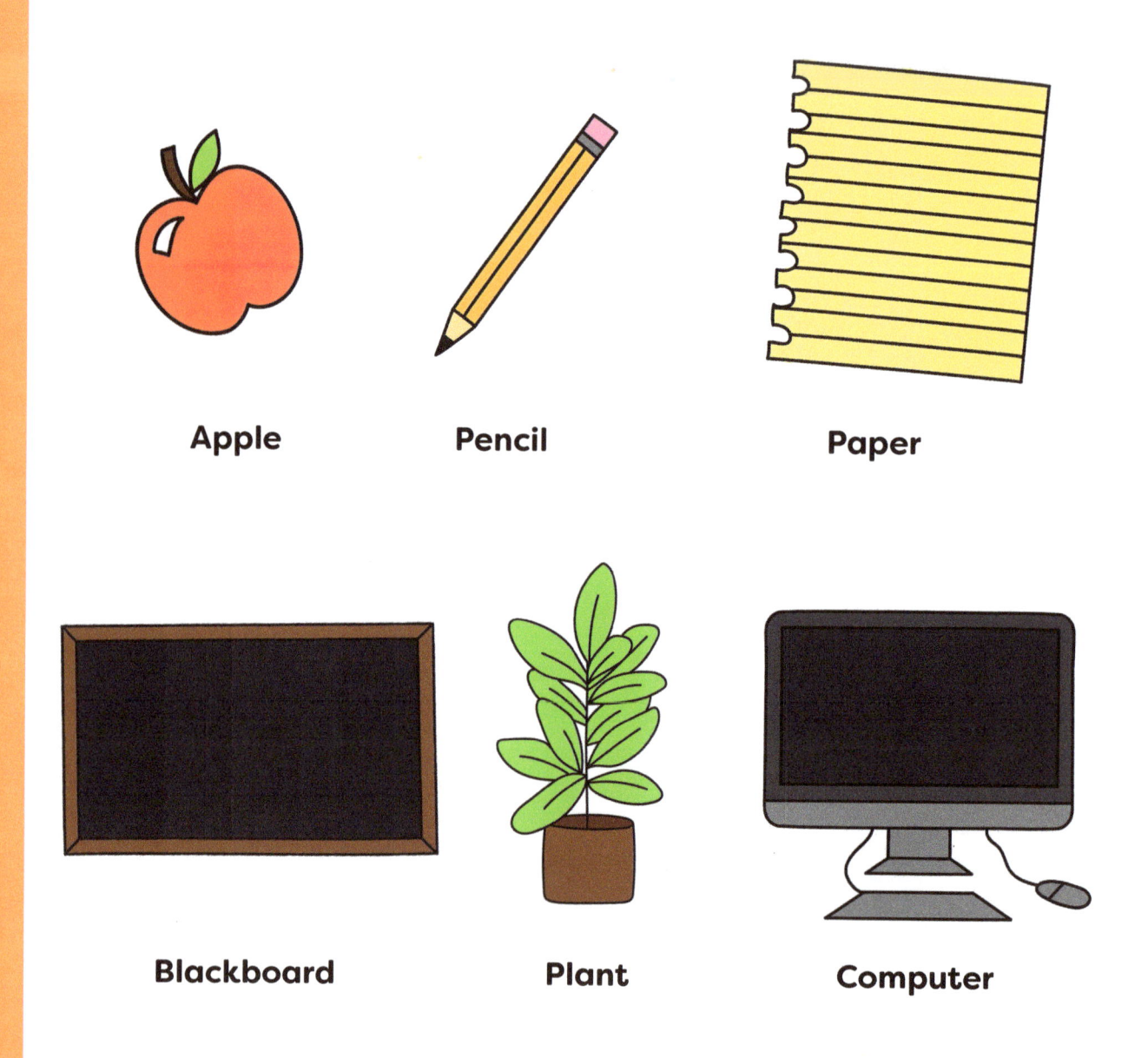

Apple   **Pencil**   **Paper**

Blackboard   **Plant**   **Computer**

GEOLOGY ACTIVITY BOOK FOR KIDS

GEOLOGY IN ACTION

In this "explosive" experiment, you'll make chalk art with baking soda, which is made from the mineral salt. This activity is messy! Try doing it outside or in an area that's easy to clean up.

What you'll need:

2 tablespoons baking soda	1 cup cornstarch
1 square of toilet paper	1 cup vinegar
Plastic zipper storage bag	Food coloring

What to do:

1. Pour the baking soda in the center of the toilet paper square. Wrap the paper around to create a ball. Set aside.

2. Fill the bag with the cornstarch, vinegar, and five drops of the food coloring.

3. Seal the bag. Shake it to mix.

4. Open the bag. Quickly toss the baking soda ball into the bag and seal it.

5. Place the bag on the ground. Step back and watch it explode!

GEOLOGY IN THE CLASSROOM

Rock Around the House:
Geology at Home

Rocks and minerals are also part of life at home. Rocks and minerals are used for cooking, cleaning, and playing. They are also used to bring electricity to your home. A lot of the things you do every day would not be possible without rocks and minerals!

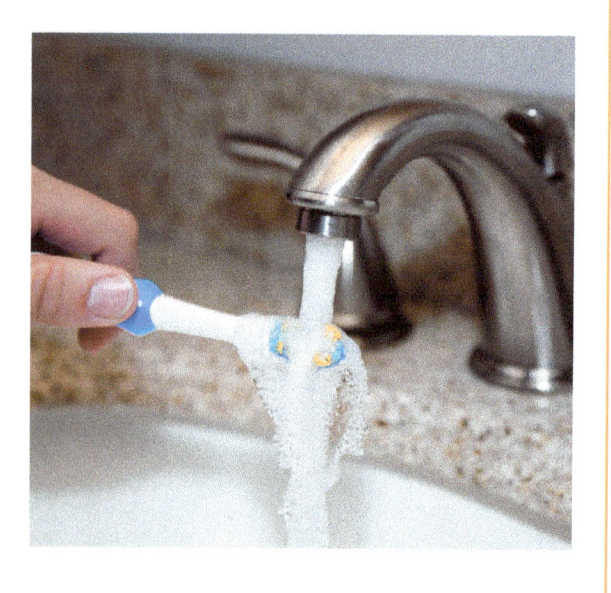

5 FUN FACTS

1. Your bathroom is full of rocks and minerals. A mineral called talc is used to make deodorant. A rock called limestone is in toothpaste.

2. Minerals help make food taste good! Salt is a mineral used in cooking.

3. Many people swallow zinc, a mineral, to help prevent sickness.

4. It takes many minerals to make a video game console, including gold.

5. Coal is a rock used to make electricity. The electrical wires are made from a mineral called silver.

ACTIVITY

Each household item in the word search is made from rocks and minerals. Can you find all the words? Be sure to look for words that go side to side and up and down!

Countertop **Electronics** **Tools**

Deodorant **Jewelry** **Toothpaste**

Electricity **Makeup** **Wires**

Mirrors

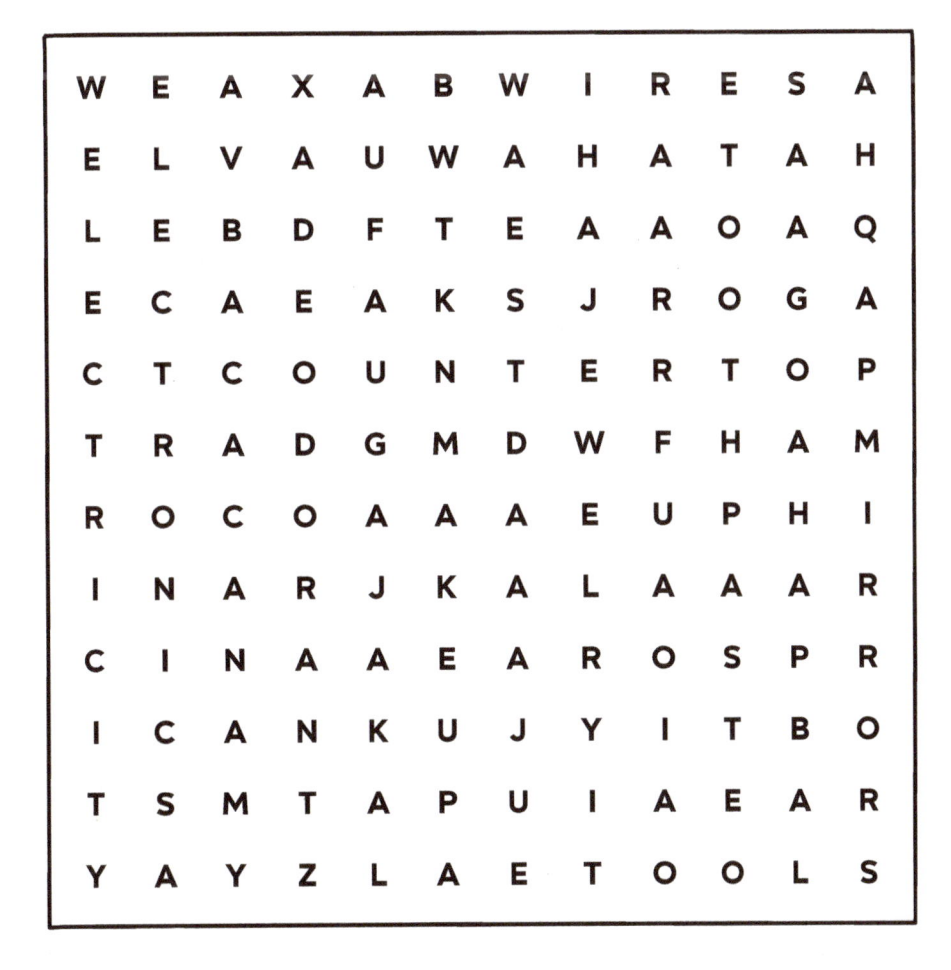

W	E	A	X	A	B	W	I	R	E	S	A
E	L	V	A	U	W	A	H	A	T	A	H
L	E	B	D	F	T	E	A	A	O	A	Q
E	C	A	E	A	K	S	J	R	O	G	A
C	T	C	O	U	N	T	E	R	T	O	P
T	R	A	D	G	M	D	W	F	H	A	M
R	O	C	O	A	A	A	E	U	P	H	I
I	N	A	R	J	K	A	L	A	A	A	R
C	I	N	A	A	E	A	R	O	S	P	R
I	C	A	N	K	U	J	Y	I	T	B	O
T	S	M	T	A	P	U	I	A	E	A	R
Y	A	Y	Z	L	A	E	T	O	O	L	S

GEOLOGY AT HOME   23

GEOLOGY IN ACTION

Let's look for more rocks and minerals in your everyday life!

What you'll need:

Magazines or catalogs

Scissors

Glue

1 sheet of construction paper

Internet

What to do:

1. Look through several magazines and catalogs. Being careful with sharp scissors, cut out images of objects made from rocks and minerals that are part of your daily life. Find at least five images.

2. Glue the images to the construction paper to create a collage.

3. Have an adult help you look up each item on the internet to see what it is made of. What rocks and minerals make up each object?

4. Share your collage with others.

Crystal Clear:
Crystal Shapes and Structures

Have you ever seen a rock that sparkled? The sparkly parts in rocks are crystals. The materials that form crystals create unique patterns. The pattern of the materials determines the shape of the crystal. Crystals come in seven shapes.

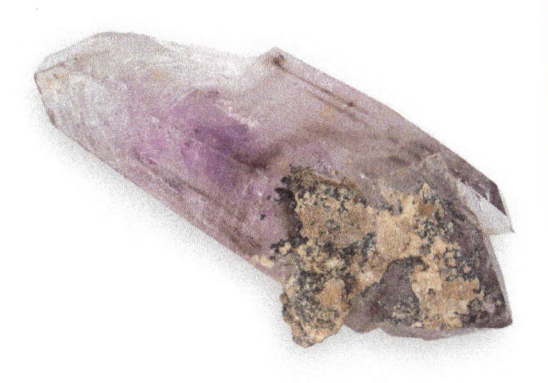

AMETHYST CRYSTALS ARE PURPLE AND HAVE SIX SIDES.

5 FUN FACTS

1. Crystals are made in different ways. Some are made when hot liquids cool. Others form when water disappears, leaving minerals behind.

2. Snowflakes are ice crystals.

3. Crystals grow bigger over time.

4. Some of the world's largest crystals were found in an underwater cave in Mexico. The crystals weighed 55 tons. That's heavier than 27 cars!

5. Some computer screens, called LCD screens, use liquid crystals to show images.

ACTIVITY

Connect the dots to take a closer look at four crystal shapes. Sound out the name of each crystal shape as you connect the dots.

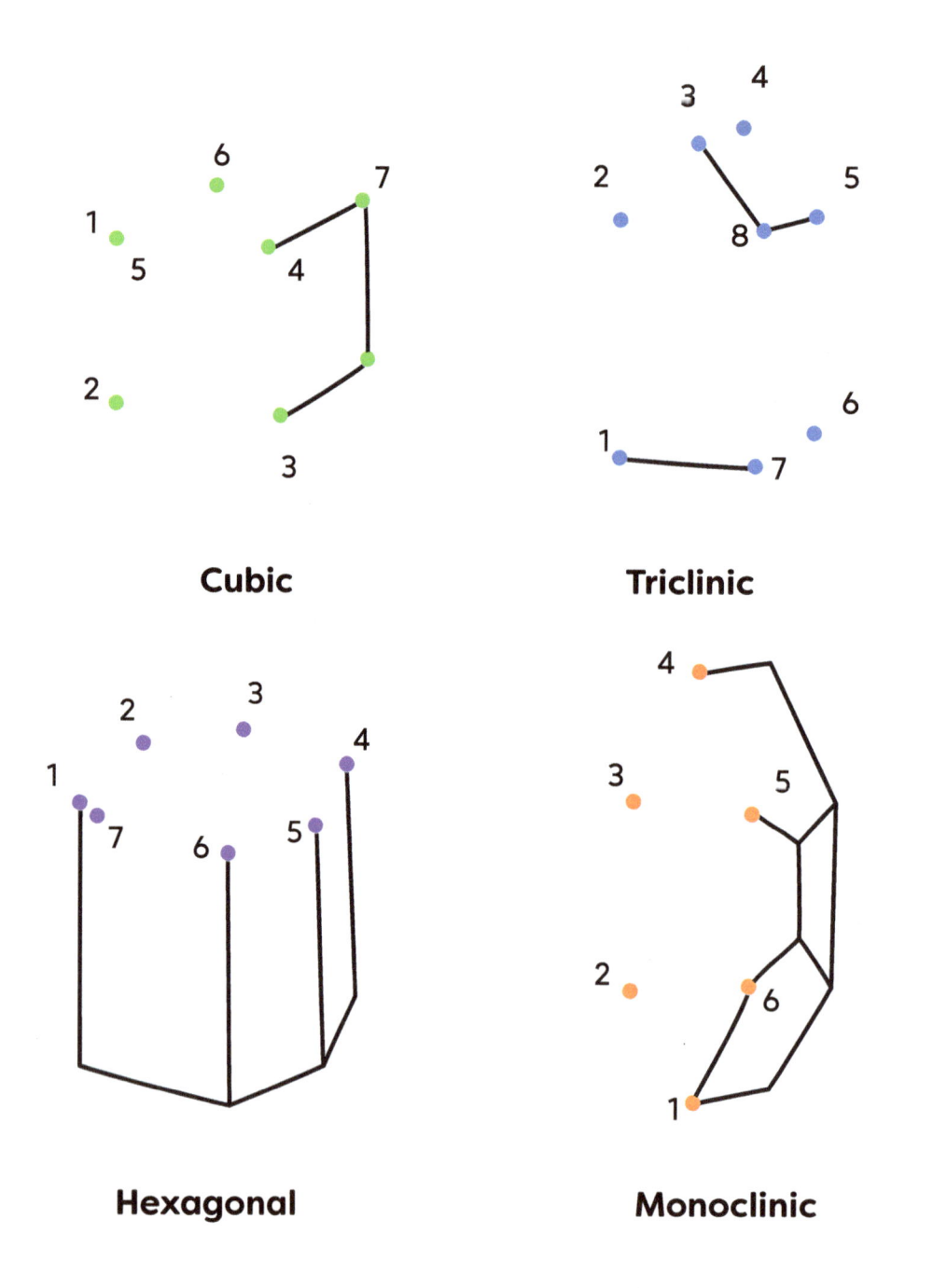

Cubic

Triclinic

Hexagonal

Monoclinic

26 GEOLOGY ACTIVITY BOOK FOR KIDS

GEOLOGY IN ACTION

It's easy to grow your own crystals at home!

What you'll need:

4 cups water

Large glass jar

2 cups borax

Spoon

Pipe cleaner

Pencil

What to do:

1. Ask an adult to help you heat up the water. Pour the hot water into the glass jar.

2. Add the borax and stir with the spoon.

3. Wrap one end of the pipe cleaner around the center of the pencil.

4. Set the pencil across the top of the jar, so the pipe cleaner hangs down into the liquid. Set the jar aside for three days.

5. Check the jar. What do you find? What shape are the crystals?

What's Inside a Rock:
Geodes

From the outside, some candy bars look like they are only chocolate. When you bite into them, though, you find they are filled with other things like caramel and peanuts. Some rocks are the same way! They look plain but are filled with crystals on the inside. These crystal-filled rocks are called geodes.

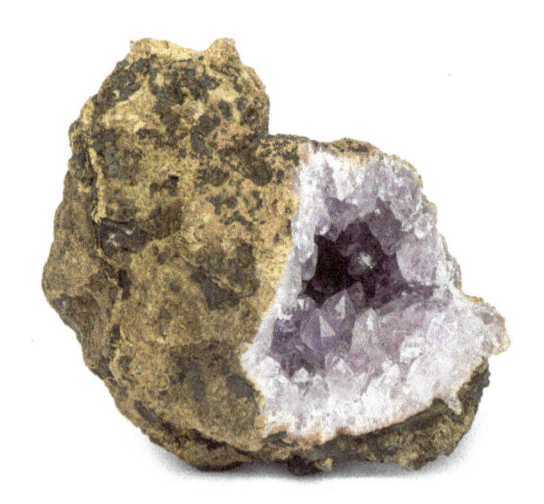

AMETHYST CRYSTALS CAN FORM INSIDE GEODES. WHAT A BEAUTIFUL SURPRISE!

5 FUN FACTS

1. Geodes are made in the open space inside a rock. Water pours in and leaves behind minerals that form crystals.

2. The bigger the crystals, the older the geode.

3. The color of a geode depends on the minerals that formed it.

4. Two common crystals in geodes are quartz and amethyst. Pure quartz is colorless. Amethyst is purple.

5. The best places to find geodes are in deserts and near volcanoes.

ACTIVITY

Use the key to color the geode. Can you tell what type of crystal is inside the rock?

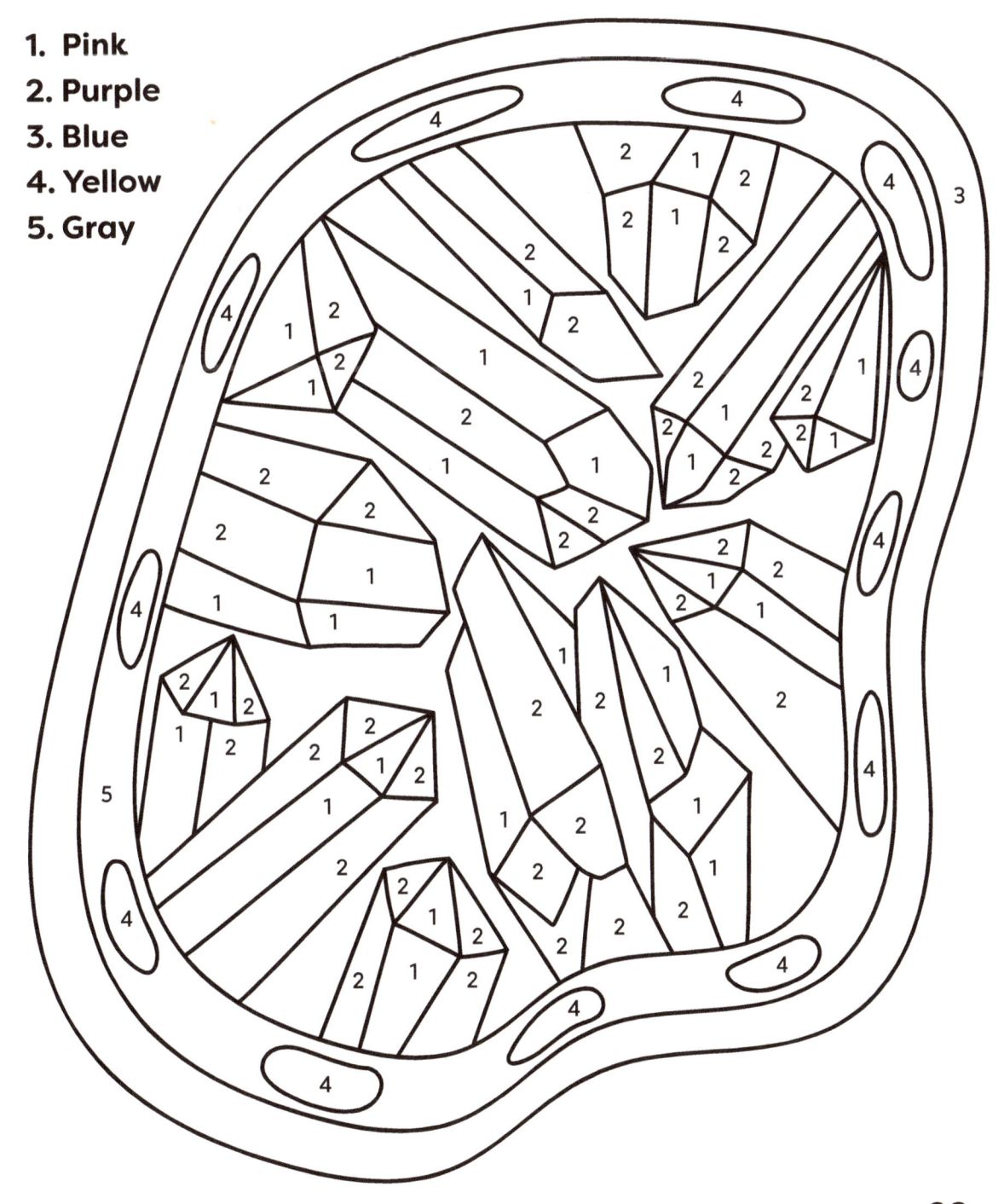

1. Pink
2. Purple
3. Blue
4. Yellow
5. Gray

GEODES **29**

GEOLOGY IN ACTION

You can't always find geodes in your backyard. These crystal-filled rocks are found in only a few places around the world. But you can grow your geodes in your kitchen.

What you'll need:

1 egg

2 cups water

2 glass jars

Spoon

½ cup borax

Food coloring

What to do:

1. Carefully crack the egg in half. Discard the egg but save the shell. Gently rinse the remaining egg off the shell.

2. Ask an adult to heat up the water. Split the hot water between the glass jars.

3. Use the spoon to quickly stir the borax and five drops of the food coloring into each jar.

4. Put half of a shell, with the inside facing up, inside each of the jars. Set aside for three days.

5. Check the jars. What do you find? What colors are your geodes?

Pretty Precious:
Gems and Gemstones

Gemstones are rocks and minerals that are cut and polished so that they look shiny and beautiful. They often make gorgeous jewelry. Diamonds, rubies, sapphires, and emeralds are **precious gemstones**. They are called precious because they are rare and expensive. All other gems are called **semiprecious gemstones**.

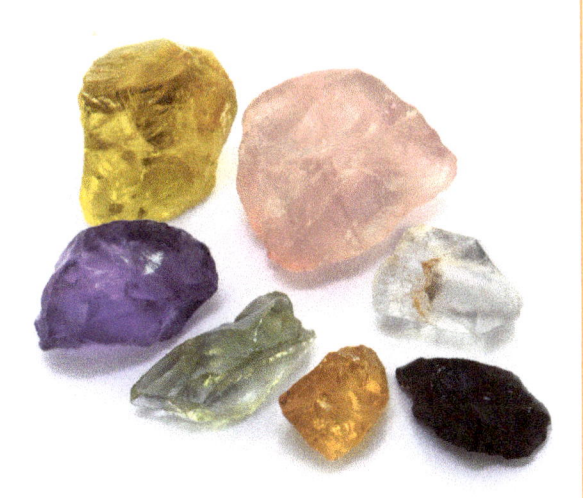

GEMSTONES CAN BE MANY COLORS, LIKE PINK ROSE QUARTZ AND ORANGE CITRINE.

5 FUN FACTS

1. Diamonds are the hardest material on Earth.

2. It takes one to three years to grow a pearl.

3. Alexandrite is a color-changing gemstone. It is green in sunlight and red in lamplight.

4. Amber is the lightest gemstone. It is so light that it can float in salt water.

5. Gemstones are weighed using a measurement called carats.

ACTIVITY

Find each of the semiprecious gemstones hidden in the word search. Be sure to look for words that go side to side and up and down!

Alexandrite	**Jade**	**Pearl**
Amber	**Moonstone**	**Tanzanite**
Aquamarine	**Onyx**	**Topaz**
Garnet	**Opal**	**Turquoise**

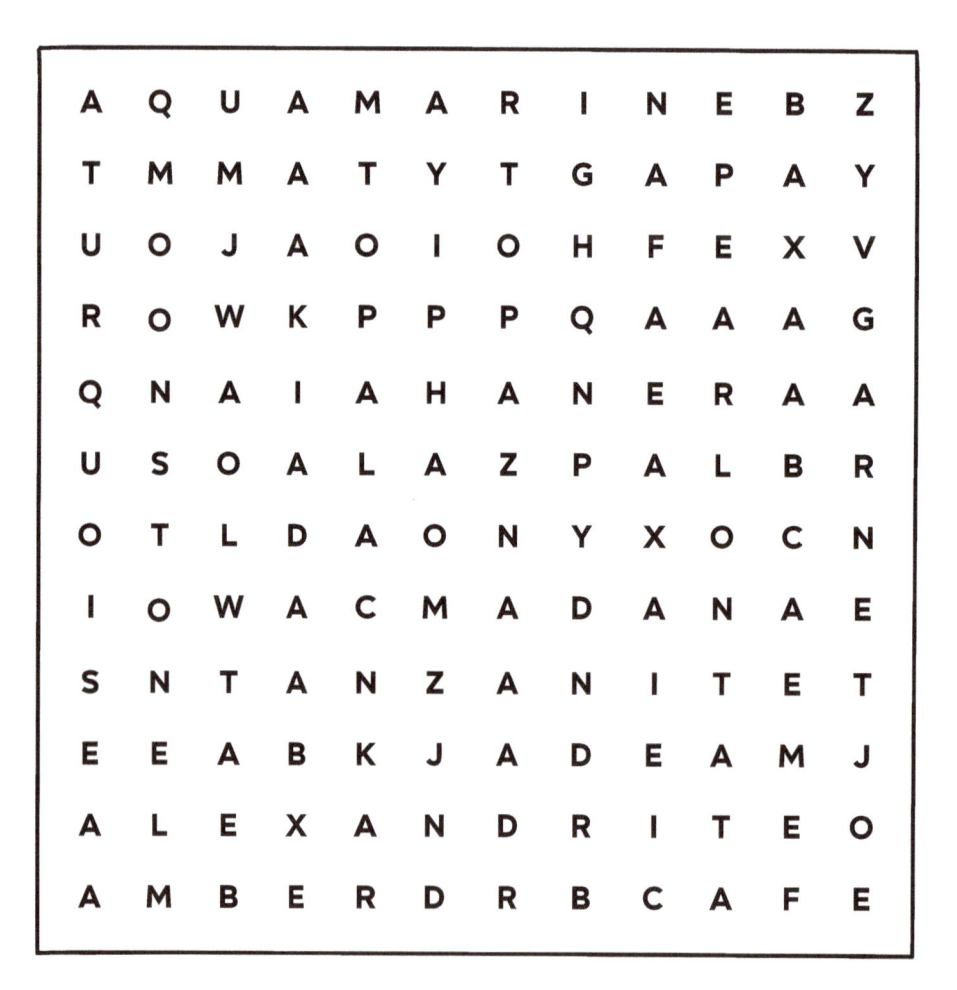

A	Q	U	A	M	A	R	I	N	E	B	Z
T	M	M	A	T	Y	T	G	A	P	A	Y
U	O	J	A	O	I	O	H	F	E	X	V
R	O	W	K	P	P	P	Q	A	A	A	G
Q	N	A	I	A	H	A	N	E	R	A	A
U	S	O	A	L	A	Z	P	A	L	B	R
O	T	L	D	A	O	N	Y	X	O	C	N
I	O	W	A	C	M	A	D	A	N	A	E
S	N	T	A	N	Z	A	N	I	T	E	T
E	E	A	B	K	J	A	D	E	A	M	J
A	L	E	X	A	N	D	R	I	T	E	O
A	M	B	E	R	D	R	B	C	A	F	E

32 GEOLOGY ACTIVITY BOOK FOR KIDS

GEOLOGY IN ACTION

Inside the Earth, it can take millions of years to form gems! But you can make your own gems at home in just a few days.

What you'll need:

1 cup rock salt

Plastic zipper storage bag

Food coloring

Baking sheet

Medium bowl

¼ cup glue

1 sheet of parchment paper

What to do:

1. Pour the rock salt into the plastic bag. Add 10 drops of the food coloring. Seal the bag. Shake to completely cover the rock salt in the food coloring.

2. Pour the contents of the bag onto the baking sheet to dry. Allow to dry for one hour or until you can touch the salt without it leaving color on your fingers.

3. Once dry, pour the colored salt into the bowl. Add the glue. Mix with your hands until you can form small balls.

4. Put the balls on the parchment paper to dry for two days. Based on the color, what type of gems did you make?

Happy Birthday:
Birthstones

Every person has their own special gem that tells when they were born. These gems are called birthstones. Every month has a birthstone. People wear these gems as jewelry to share and celebrate the month in which they were born. What is your birthstone?

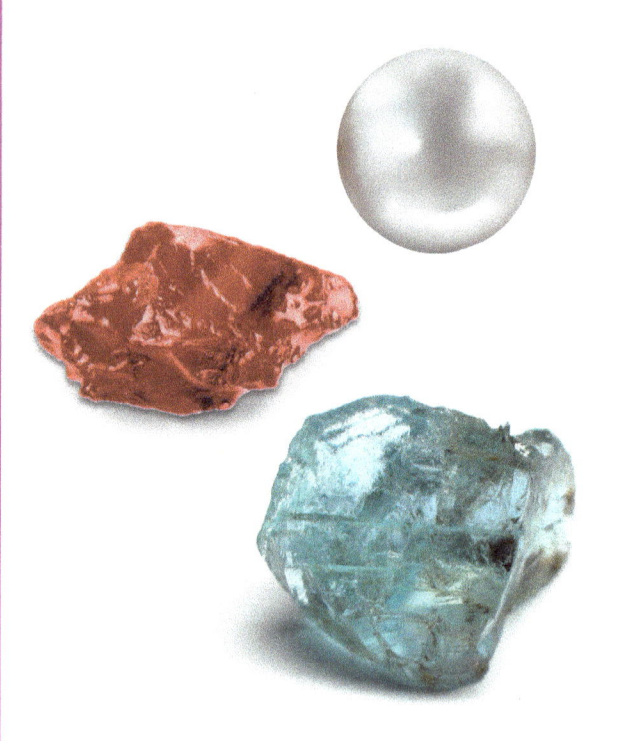

PEARL, RUBY, AND AQUAMARINE ARE ALL BIRTHSTONES.

5 FUN FACTS

1. The idea of birthstones has been around for thousands of years.

2. People used to believe that birthstones had power. They said garnet could stop bad dreams.

3. Some cultures believe that wearing your birthstone makes you stronger.

4. Long ago, kings and queens wore sapphires. They believed the gems would protect them from disloyal people.

5. Opal is said to be the most magical birthstone because it is so colorful.

ACTIVITY

Complete the birthstone chart by coloring each gem the correct color.

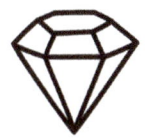

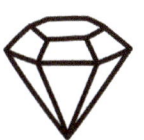

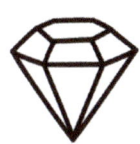

January
Garnet: Red

February
Amethyst: Purple

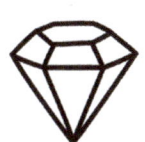

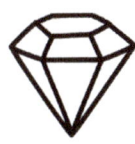

March
Bloodstone: Dark green with red or orange spots

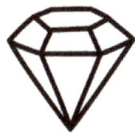

April
Diamond: Clear

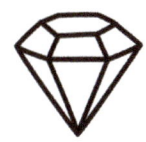

May
Emerald: Dark green

June
Pearl: White

July
Ruby: Dark red

August
Onyx: Black

September
Sapphire: Dark blue

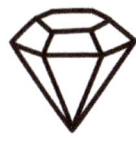

October
Opal: White with some blue, yellow, pink, and purple

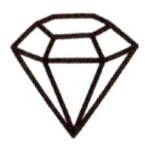

November
Topaz: Yellow-orange

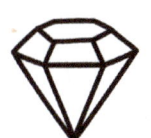

December
Turquoise: Blue-green

GEOLOGY IN ACTION

Buying birthstone jewelry can be expensive, but you can easily re-create birthstone jewelry at home using beads.

What you'll need:

Elastic cord

Scissors

Beads (the color of your birthstone)

What to do:

1. Wrap the elastic cord around your wrist. Ask an adult to help you cut the cord with scissors so that it is slightly bigger than your wrist.

2. String the beads on the elastic cord.

3. Ask an adult to tie the bracelet around your wrist.

4. Use your bracelet to tell others about birthstones.

Fantastic Planet:
Fossils

Have you ever found a rock that looks like a plant was printed on it? If so, you've discovered a fossil! Fossils are the remains of ancient plants and animals. Fossils teach us about Earth's past. Fossils found in rocks teach us what plants and animals existed when the rock formed.

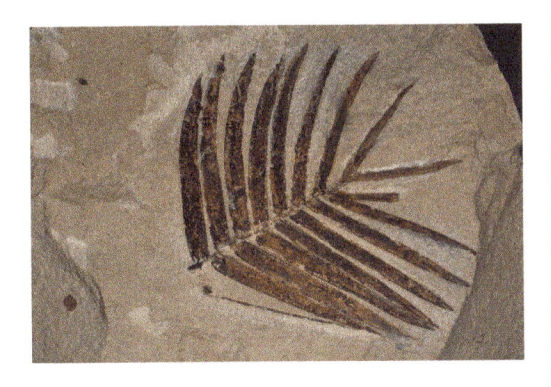

FOSSILS LIKE THIS ONE HELP US KNOW WHAT PLANTS AND ANIMALS LOOKED LIKE LONG AGO.

5 FUN FACTS

1. An item must be more than 10,000 years old to be a fossil.

2. Bones and teeth, footprints, eggs, and poop are all examples of fossils.

3. Fossils take a long time to find. It took 28 years to dig out the bones of a dinosaur in Antarctica.

4. Scientists found the bones of a giant parrot that lived millions of years ago. They named the bird Squawkzilla.

5. "Fossilized poop" once sold for more than $10,000. Later, scientists learned it wasn't actually poop. It was just minerals.

ACTIVITY

Is there a fossil hidden in this rock? Connect the dots to find out.

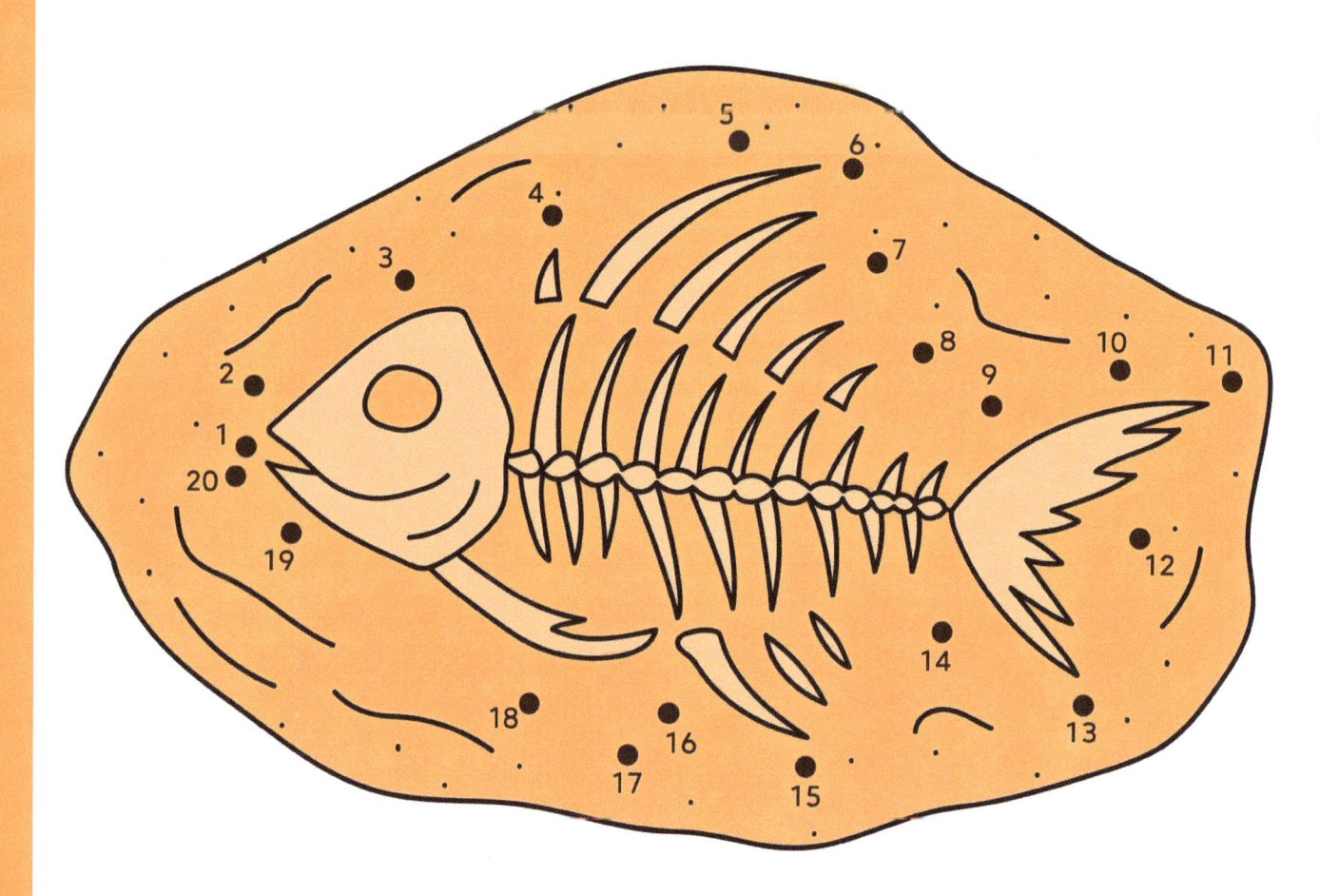

38 GEOLOGY ACTIVITY BOOK FOR KIDS

GEOLOGY IN ACTION

In this fun activity, you will create fossil models using food.

What you'll need:

8 slices of bread

6 gummy worms

1 (18-inch-long) sheet of plastic wrap

Heavy books

What to do:

1. Stack two slices of the bread on top of the plastic wrap.

2. Put two gummy worms, spaced out, on top of the bread.

3. Keep layering two slices of the bread and two gummy worms until all of the bread is used.

4. Wrap the stack in the plastic wrap. Lay several heavy books on top.

5. Let the stack sit on the counter for two hours, then remove the books. Slowly peel back each layer of the bread. What do you find?

Shake It Up:
Earthquakes

The Earth's surface is like a giant puzzle. It is broken into large pieces called **tectonic plates**. These plates are always moving under your feet. Normally, you can't feel them moving because they move so slowly. But sometimes these plates grind against each other, which creates earthquakes.

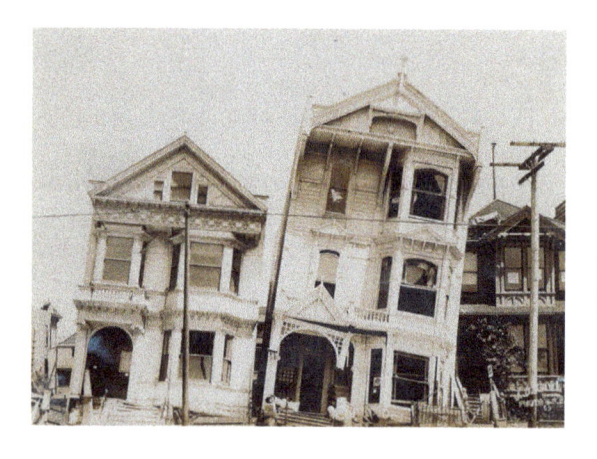

IN 1906, A LARGE EARTHQUAKE SHOOK SAN FRANCISCO.

5 FUN FACTS

1. Earth's surface is made of seven large tectonic plates and many small tectonic plates. Tectonic plates form the continents and the solid surface at the bottom of the ocean.

2. Most earthquakes happen along the edges of tectonic plates.

3. Underwater earthquakes can create large waves called **tsunamis**. Tsunamis can be as tall as buildings.

4. Alaska has more earthquakes than any other state.

5. Earthquakes can happen in any type of weather.

ACTIVITY

During an earthquake, two tectonic plates grind against each other. Trace the arrows to show how the plates move during an earthquake. Then color the picture.

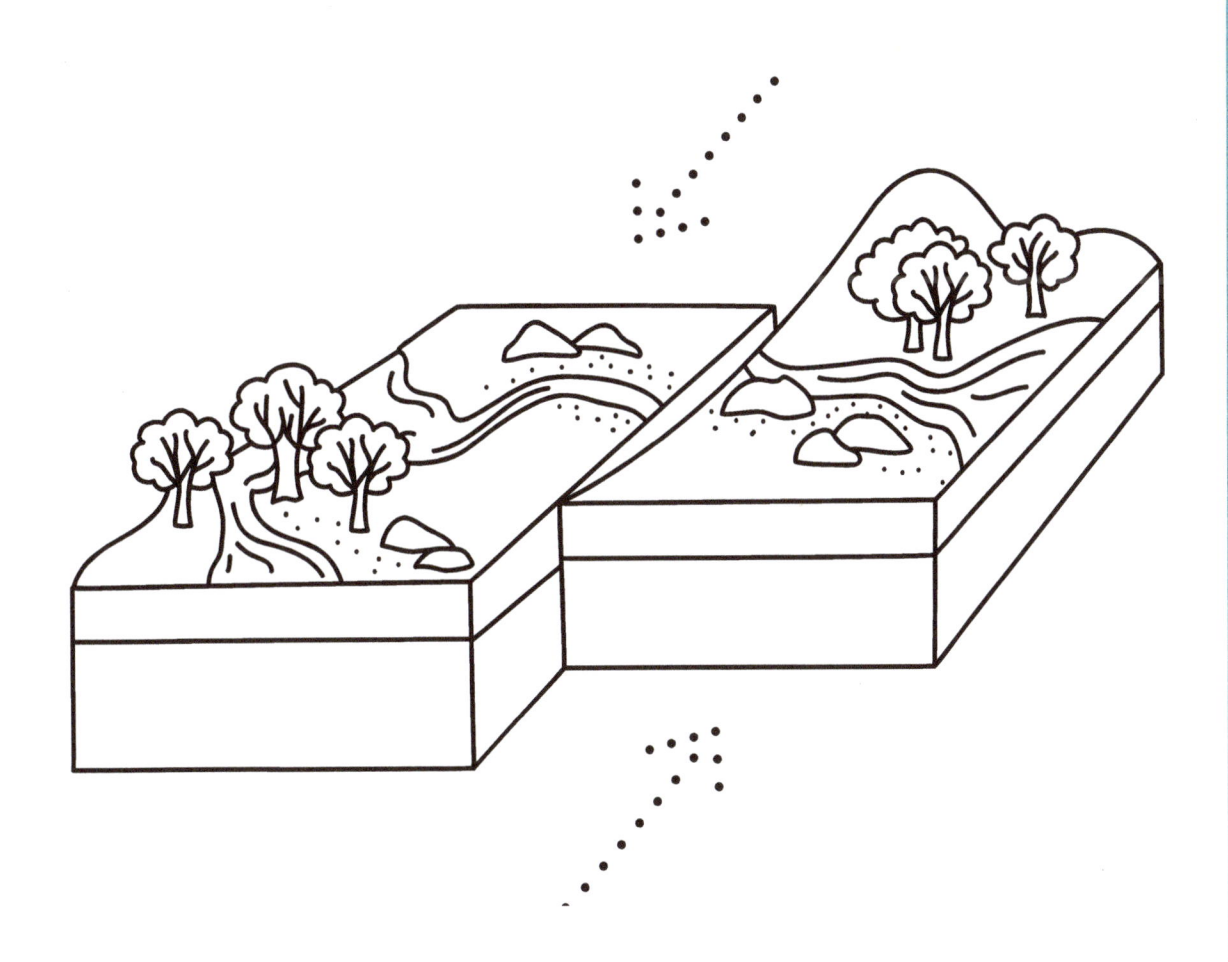

EARTHQUAKES

GEOLOGY IN ACTION

In places where earthquakes happen often, homes are built to stand even when the Earth moves. Can you create a building that survives an earthquake?

What you'll need:

1 (8- by 10-inch or larger) poster board

Toothpicks

Marshmallows

Timer or stopwatch

What to do:

1. Place the poster board on a flat, solid surface.

2. Construct your building by sticking the toothpicks and marshmallows together.

3. Set the building in the center of the poster board. Put your hands on one side of the poster board. Set the timer for one minute and quickly slide the poster board back and forth.

4. Is your building still standing? Repeat the experiment several times. Try using different materials and different shapes.

Hot Lava:
Volcanoes

To understand volcanoes, it can be helpful to imagine a tea kettle. As water heats up inside the kettle, steam builds. This steam creates pressure. Eventually, the steam escapes through the spout of the kettle. This is similar to how volcanoes form. Hot magma creates steam deep within the Earth. Pressure forces the magma and steam out through cracks in the Earth.

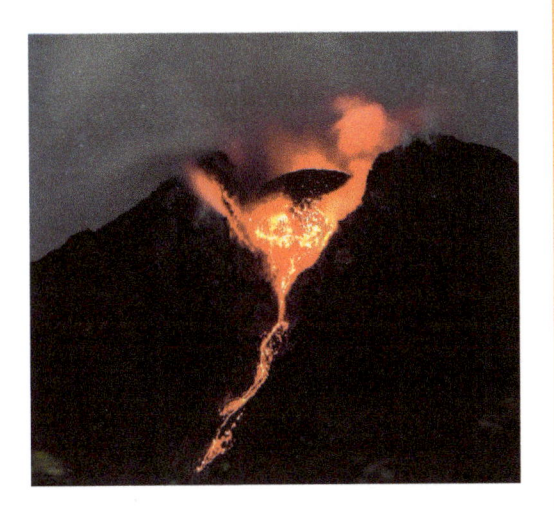

5 FUN FACTS

1. At any moment, lava is erupting from 40 to 50 volcanoes around the planet!

2. Volcanoes come in different shapes and sizes. Some look like mountains. Others look like large cracks in the Earth.

3. There are about 1,500 active volcanoes on Earth.

4. More than half of Earth's volcanoes are found around the Pacific Ocean.

5. Earth isn't the only place where volcanoes are found. Scientists have discovered volcanoes on other planets and moons, too.

ACTIVITY

Magma is building deep within the Earth. Create a volcanic eruption by completing the maze. Remember, when magma erupts from the Earth's surface, it is called lava.

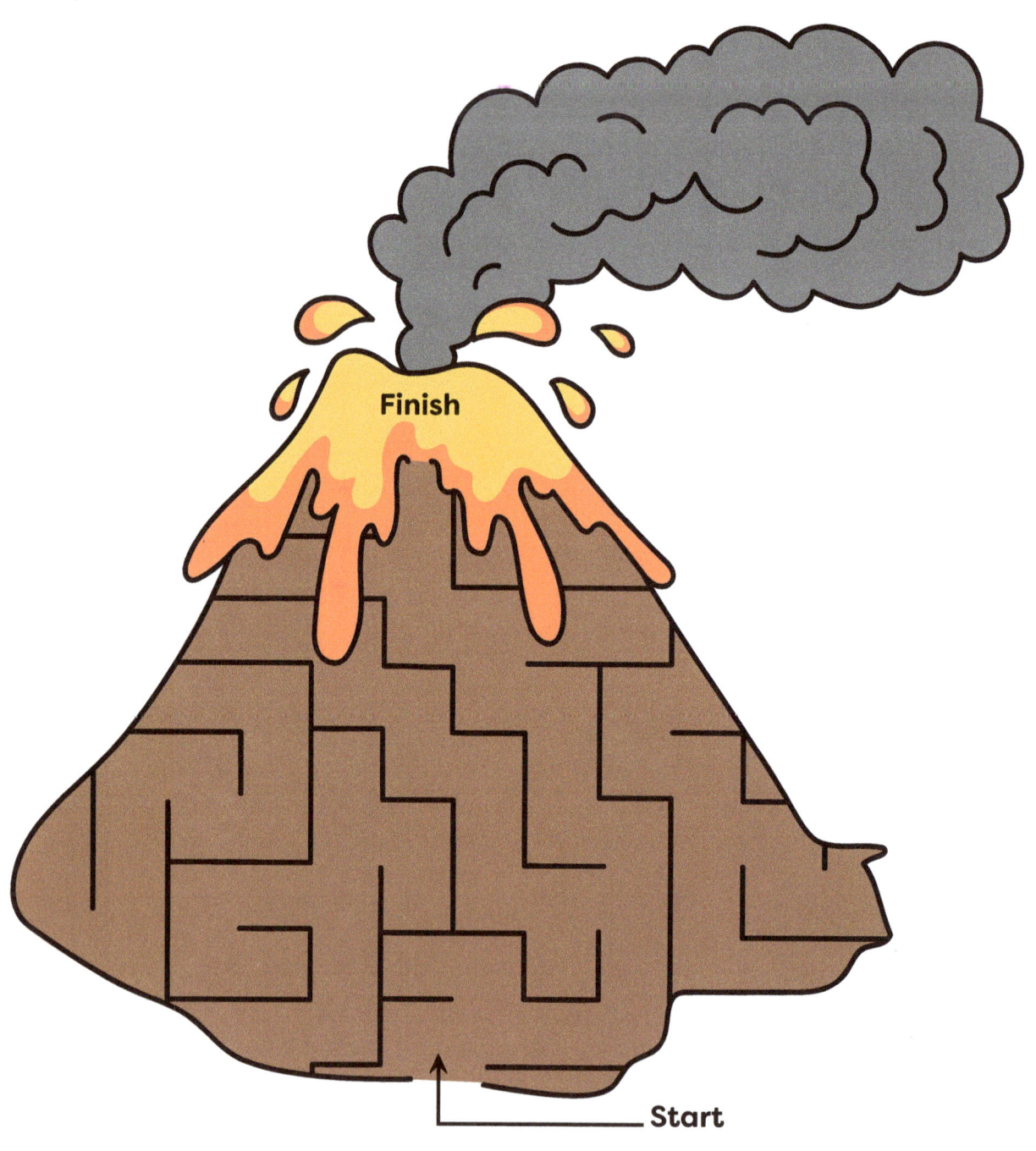

GEOLOGY IN ACTION

Let's create a volcanic eruption! Be prepared: You will get messy when your volcano explodes. It is best to complete this activity outside.

What you'll need:

Large, clear jar	**1 teaspoon dish soap**
Disposable pan	**Red food coloring**
Water	**Spoon**
5 tablespoons baking soda	**1 cup vinegar**

What to do:

1. Set the jar in the center of the pan. Fill the jar two-thirds full with the water.

2. Add the baking soda, dish soap, and six drops of the red food coloring to the jar. Mix together with the spoon.

3. Add the vinegar. Step back and watch your volcano explode!

Peak to Peak:
Mountains

Have you ever stood next to a mountain? It can make you look small. But these large landforms haven't always been so big. Mountains form as Earth's tectonic plates push into each other, slowly piling up the rocks. It takes millions of years for the rocks to become mountains.

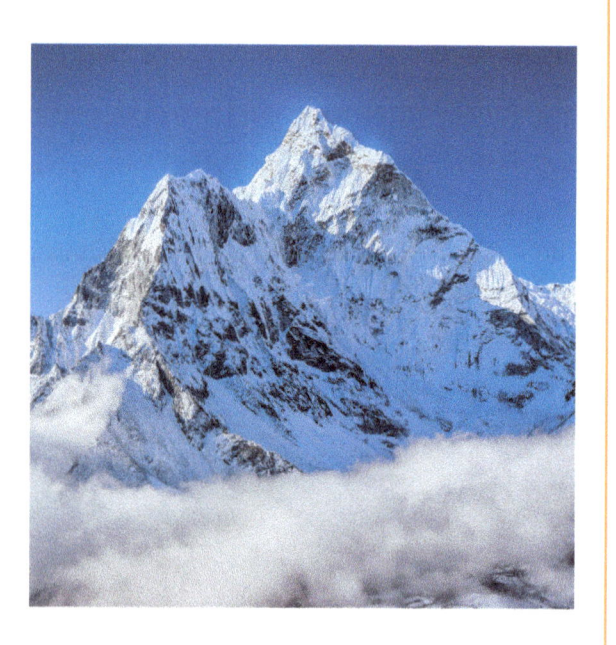

5 FUN FACTS

1. Mountains are always growing or shrinking as the tectonic plates move.

2. Mount Everest is the tallest mountain on Earth. It grows about a quarter of an inch every year.

3. The largest mountain ever discovered is on Mars. It is more than twice the size of Mount Everest.

4. A line of connected mountains is called a mountain range.

5. The largest mountain range on Earth, called the mid-ocean ridge, is below miles of ocean.

ACTIVITY

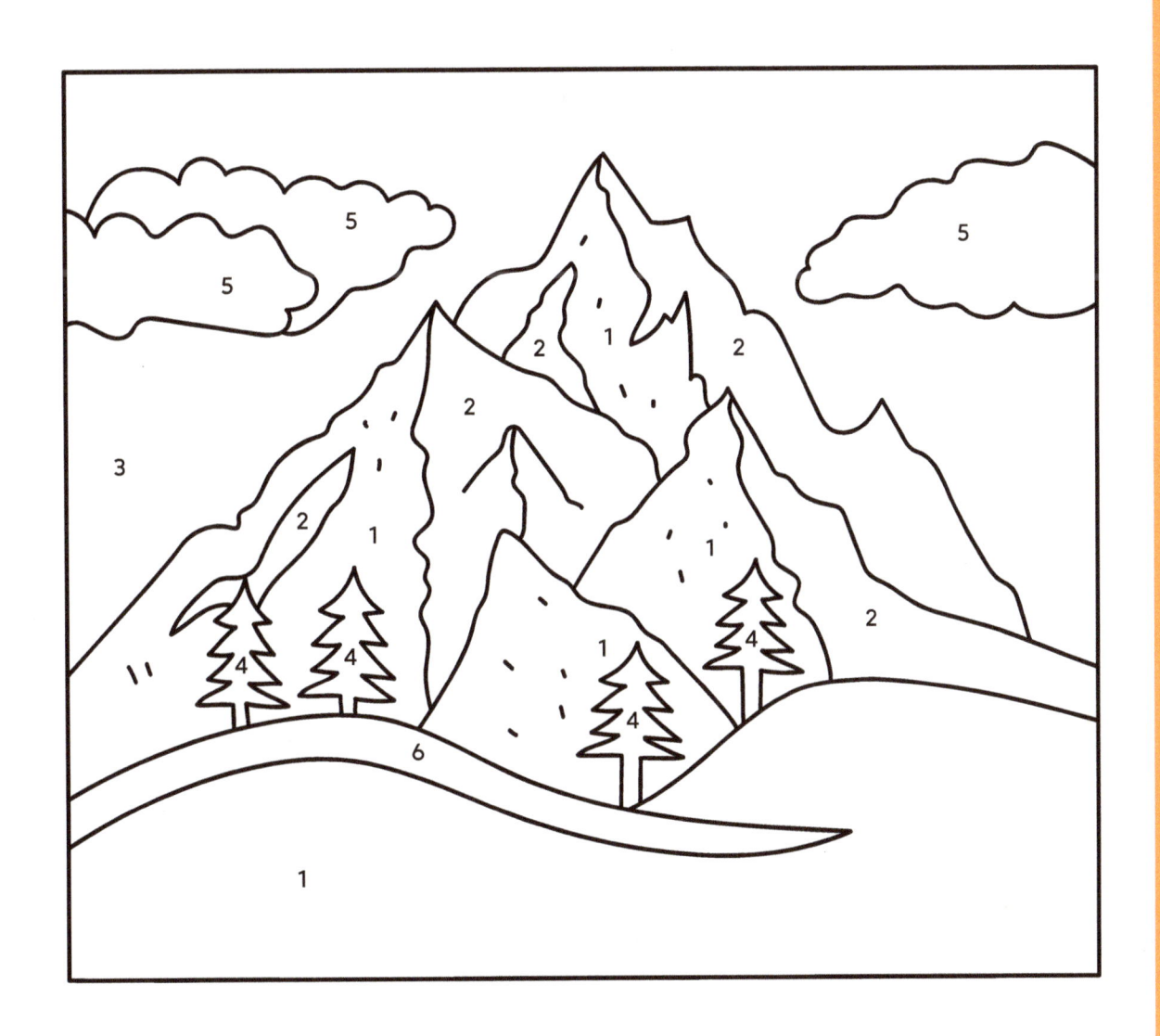

Use the key to color the mountains.

1. Gray
2. Black
3. Blue
4. Green
5. White
6. Brown

MOUNTAINS 47

GEOLOGY IN ACTION

For this edible activity, you will see how Earth's tectonic plates push together to form mountains.

What you'll need:

Plate

Whipped cream

2 graham crackers

Small bowl of water

What to do:

1. Cover the plate with a layer of the whipped cream. This represents the rocks and magma inside the Earth.

2. Dip one end of each graham cracker in the water. Hold it in the water for two seconds.

3. Lay the graham crackers next to each other on the plate with the soggy ends facing each other. These represent tectonic plates.

4. Slowly, push the graham crackers together. What happens to the graham crackers? What happens to the whipped cream?

Water, Water Everywhere:
Rivers, Streams, and Oceans

If you look at a globe, you will see more blue than green. That is because most of the Earth is covered in water. Rivers are bodies of moving water that begin uphill and move downhill until they empty into an ocean. Streams are smaller but form and move the same way. The water's movement helps shape Earth's surface.

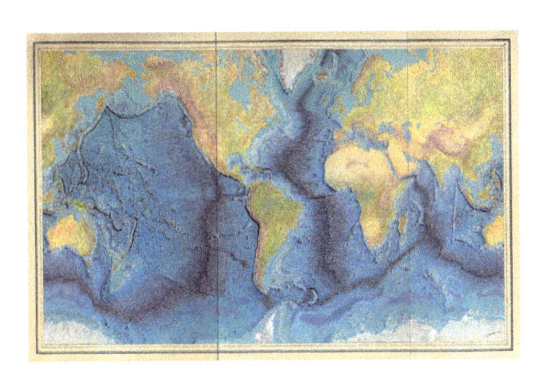

ALL THE BLUE ON THIS MAP IS WATER! ALL THE GREEN AND BROWN IS LAND. DO YOU SEE MORE LAND, OR MORE WATER?

5 FUN FACTS

1. Most rivers are made of melting snow or glaciers.

2. Rivers come in many colors. They can be blue, brown, black, yellow, or red. The plants and soil surrounding a river change its color.

3. If you drag a fork over butter, it leaves a mark. The same thing happens when water runs over Earth's surface.

4. Rivers and streams flow into the oceans, and all the oceans flow into one another.

5. Almost all of Earth's water is salt water. That means it can't be used for drinking.

ACTIVITY

Can you find all of the water features? Color the rivers blue. Color the ocean purple.

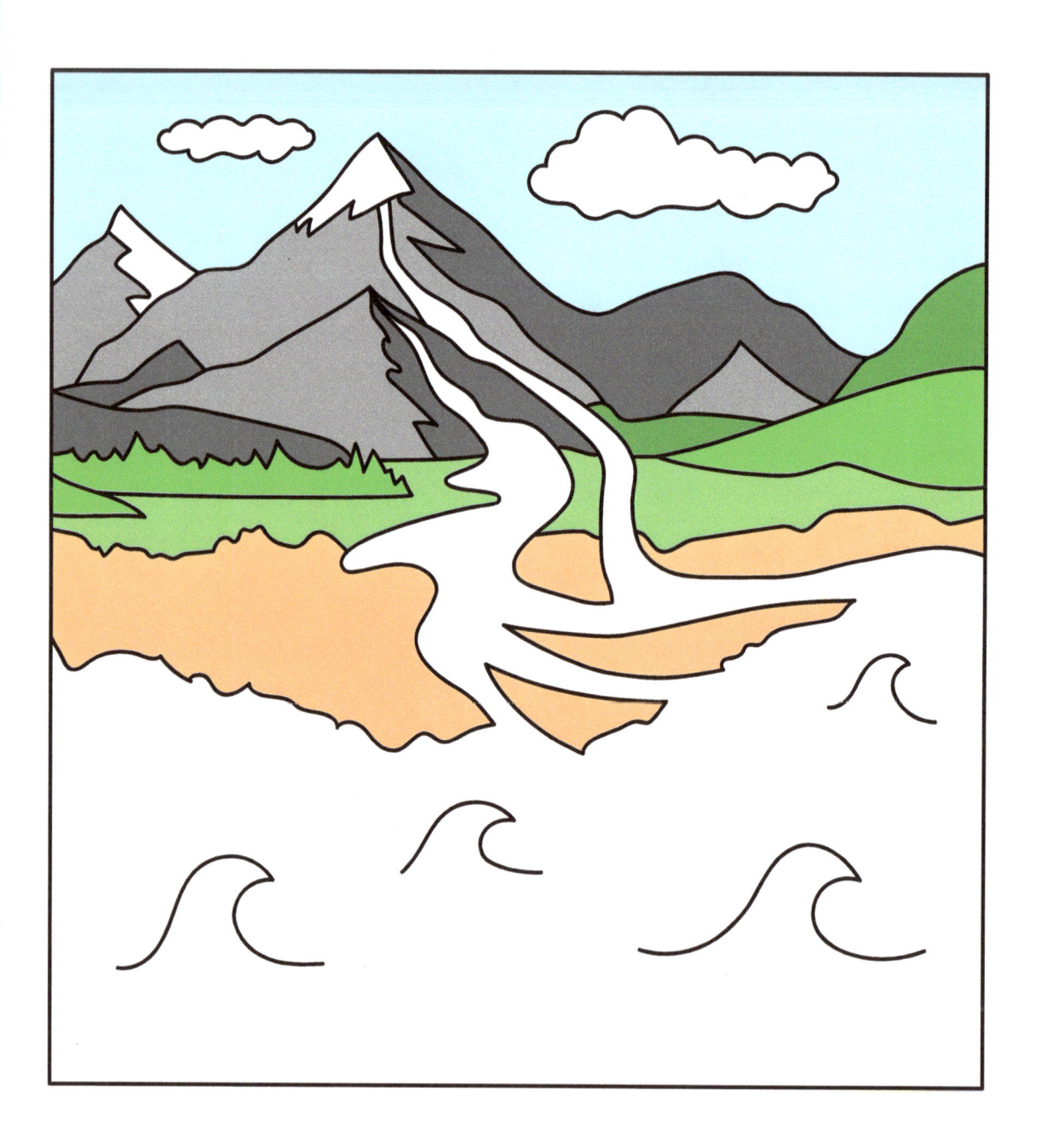

GEOLOGY IN ACTION

Get wet as you model how water moves across the land! It is best to complete this activity outside.

What you'll need:

1 (8½- by 11-inch) sheet of paper

Blue marker or pen

Spray bottle filled with water

What to do:

1. Crumple and uncrumple the paper. Some parts will be raised. Those are mountains.

2. Using the marker or pen, draw a path on the paper that you think the water will follow.

3. Hold the spray bottle about one foot away from the paper. Spray the paper three times.

4. Watch carefully to see how the water runs. Did it follow the path you created? Which parts of the model represent rivers?

RIVERS, STREAMS, AND OCEANS

Wet and Wild:
Weathering

What happens if you hit glass with a hammer? It breaks into smaller parts! The same thing happens to rocks when they are hit by wind or water. Weathering occurs when rocks and soil are broken into sediments. Wind, water, ice, and living things cause weathering. For example, wind blowing across a mountain breaks off small rocks. Over time, the mountain changes shape.

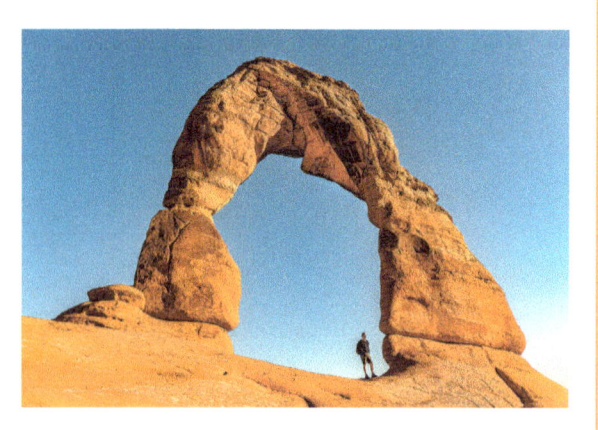

DELICATE ARCH WAS FORMED AS WIND, WATER, AND ICE SLOWLY WASHED AWAY OR BROKE OFF PIECES OF THE ROCK.

5 FUN FACTS

1. Weathering can carve arches, caves, and holes into mountains.

2. Rocks inside the Earth can be weathered by water inside the Earth.

3. Rain slowly dissolves rocks.

4. In the desert, rocks get bigger in the day when it is hot. Rocks get smaller at night when it is cold. The temperature changes cause the rocks to break into sediments.

5. Weathering happens faster in places where it gets very hot or very cold.

ACTIVITY

Match the images to show what caused the weathering. The information on pages 52 and 55 will help you find the answers.

Wind

A river

Rain

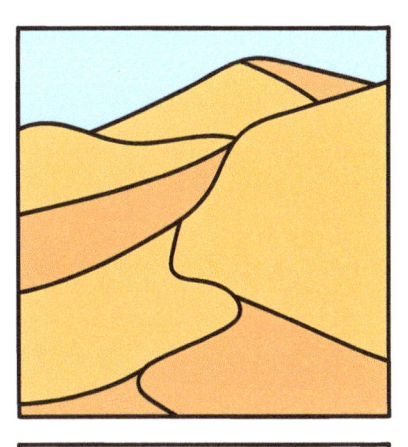

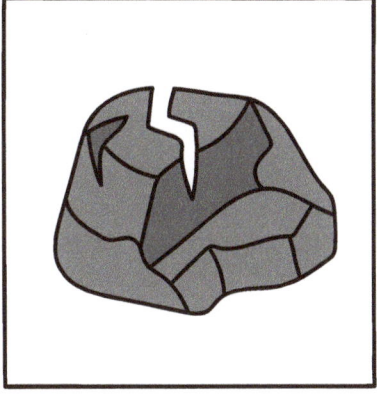

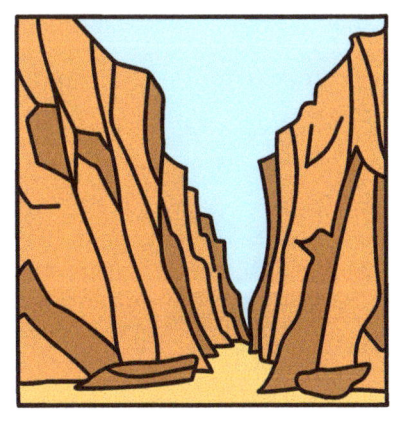

WEATHERING 53

GEOLOGY IN ACTION

Weathering happens any time rocks and soil are broken into smaller parts. In this activity, you will model weathering.

What you'll need:

4 cups water, divided

Small pot

Spoon

½ cup clear gelatin powder

Small bowl

Rocks, soil, and/or gravel

Plate

What to do:

1. Ask an adult to boil two cups of the water in the pot. Use the spoon to mix in the gelatin.

2. Fill the bowl halfway with the rocks, soil, and/or gravel.

3. Pour the gelatin mixture into the bowl to cover the rocks and soil.

4. Refrigerate the bowl overnight.

5. The next morning, turn the bowl upside down on the plate to reveal your small "mountain."

6. Ask an adult to heat the remaining two cups of water. Carefully pour the hot water over the "mountain." What happens?

Moving On:
Erosion

Think about the last time it rained. Did you notice the rain pushing rocks and dirt across the sidewalk? The process of moving sediments from one place to another is called erosion. Like weathering, erosion changes the shape of the land.

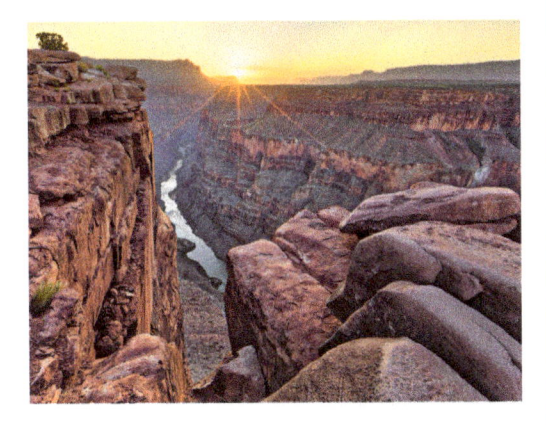

THE GRAND CANYON IS A DEEP, LONG CANYON. IMAGINE HOW MANY YEARS AND HOW MUCH WATER IT TOOK FOR A RIVER TO CARVE IT!

5 FUN FACTS

1. Wind, water, and ice are the main things that cause erosion.

2. Wind erosion has buried ancient cities. Scientists have discovered cities hidden below sand.

3. Beaches are formed by water erosion. The waves move the sand, shaping the coastlines.

4. Weathering and erosion formed the Grand Canyon. Over millions of years, a river carved the famous landform.

5. Glaciers are large pieces of moving ice. As they move, they take pieces of the land below with them. This process forms valleys.

ACTIVITY

Weathering and erosion work together to change the shape of the land. Use what you have learned on pages 52 and 55 to complete the puzzle.

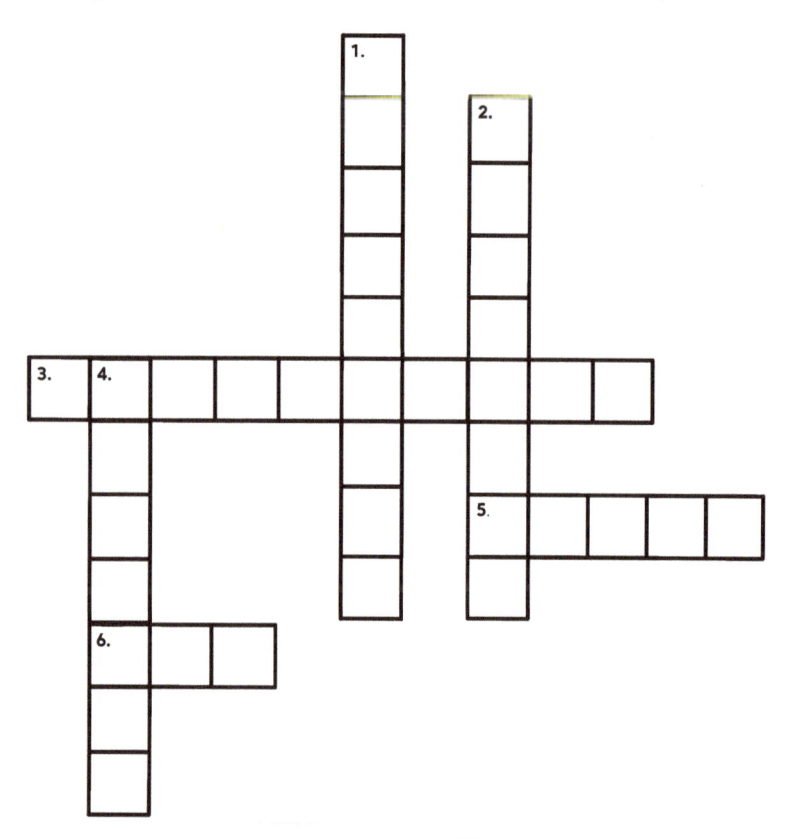

Across

3 When rocks and minerals are broken into smaller parts.

5 The Grand Canyon was formed by a _____.

6 Wind, water, and _____ cause weathering and erosion.

Down

1 Small pieces of rocks and soil.

2 Large pieces of moving ice that form valleys.

4 When sediments move from one place to another.

GEOLOGY IN ACTION

In this activity, you will use weathering and erosion to change the shape of a "mountain."

What you'll need:

10 sugar cubes

Plate

Eyedropper

Water

What to do:

1. Use the sugar cubes to build a mountain on the plate.

2. Fill the eyedropper with water.

3. Slowly drop the water on top of the mountain. Refill the eyedropper as many times as you want.

4. Does the shape of the mountain change? Explain to an adult how you modeled weathering and erosion.

Answer Key

ALL ABOUT GEOLOGY: ACTIVITY (PAGE 2)

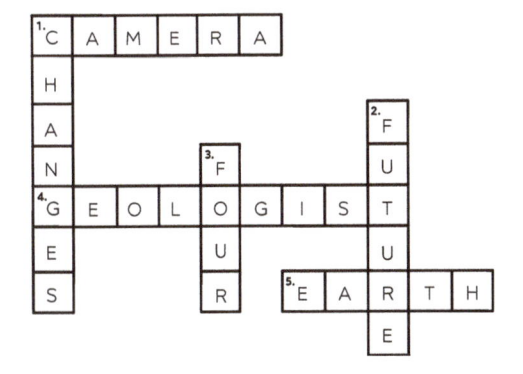

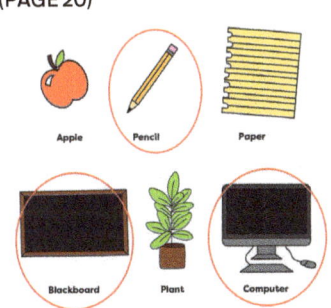

	1.C	A	M	E	R	A		
	H							
	A				2.F			
	N		3.F		U			
4.G	E	O	L	O	G	I	S	T
	E		U		T			
	S		R		U			
				5.E	A	R	T	H
					E			

HARD CORE: ACTIVITY (PAGE 5)

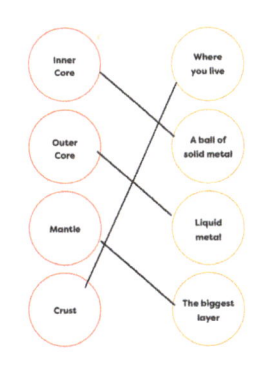

- Inner Core — A ball of solid metal
- Outer Core — Liquid metal
- Mantle — The biggest layer
- Crust — Where you live

ALL MINE: ACTIVITY (PAGE 14)

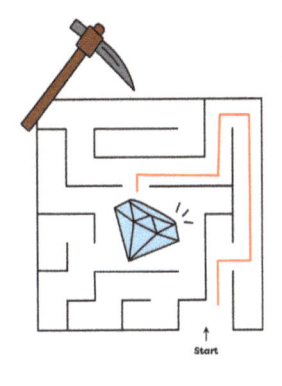

GLOW IN THE DARK: ACTIVITY (PAGE 17)

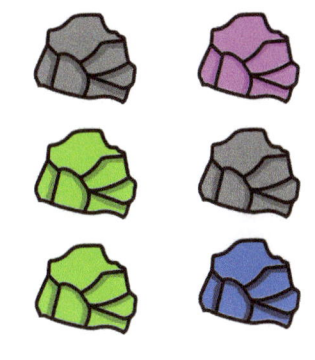

LET'S ROCK AT SCHOOL: ACTIVITY (PAGE 20)

Circled: Apple, Pencil, Paper, Blackboard, Plant, Computer

ROCK AROUND THE HOUSE: ACTIVITY (PAGE 23)

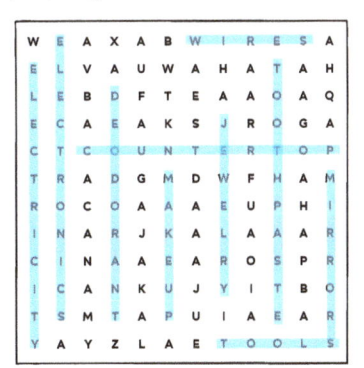

W	E	A	X	A	B	W	I	R	E	S	A
E	L	V	A	U	W	A	H	A	T	A	H
L	E	B	D	F	T	E	A	A	O	A	Q
E	C	A	E	A	K	S	J	R	O	G	A
C	T	C	O	U	N	T	E	R	T	O	P
T	R	A	D	G	M	D	W	F	H	A	M
R	O	C	O	A	A	A	E	U	P	H	I
I	N	A	R	J	K	A	L	A	A	A	R
C	I	N	A	A	E	A	R	O	S	P	R
I	C	A	N	K	U	J	Y	I	T	B	O
T	S	M	T	A	P	U	I	A	E	A	R
Y	A	Y	Z	L	A	E	T	O	O	L	S

59

CRYSTAL CLEAR:
ACTIVITY (PAGE 26)

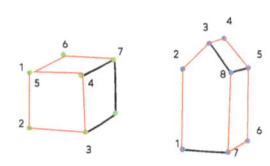

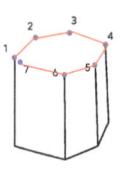

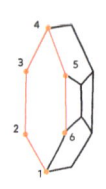

Cubic   Triclinic

Hexagonal   Monoclinic

WHAT'S INSIDE A ROCK:
ACTIVITY (PAGE 29)

ANSWER:
AMETHYST

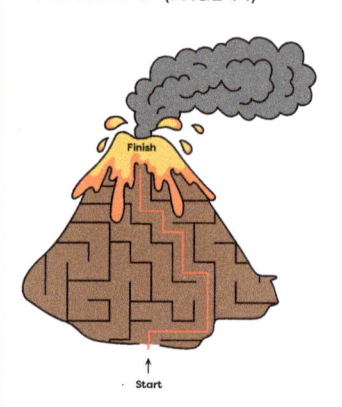

PRETTY PRECIOUS:
ACTIVITY (PAGE 32)

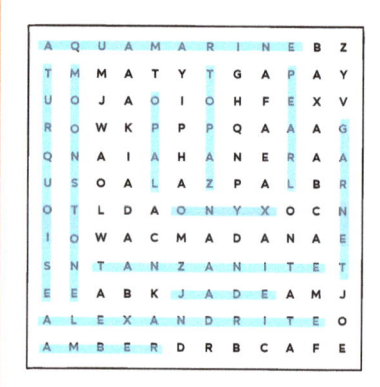

FANTASTIC PLANET:
ACTIVITY (PAGE 38):

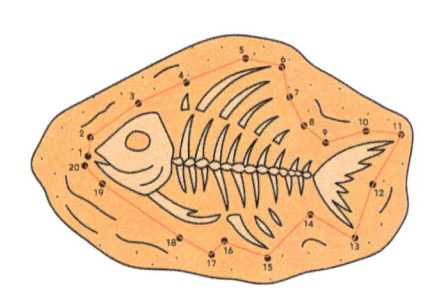

HOT LAVA:
ACTIVITY (PAGE 44)

WATER, WATER EVERYWHERE:
ACTIVITY (PAGE 50)

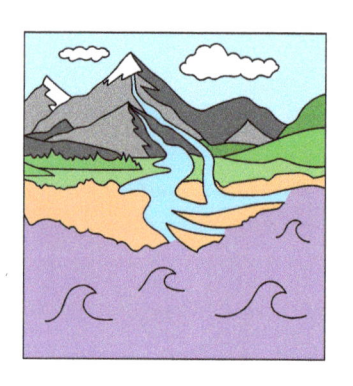

WET AND WILD:
ACTIVITY (PAGE 53)

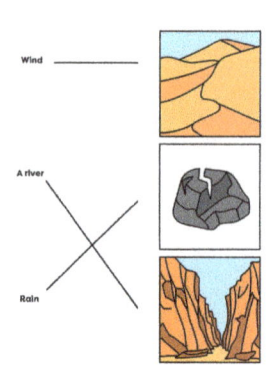

MOVING ON:
ACTIVITY (PAGE 56)

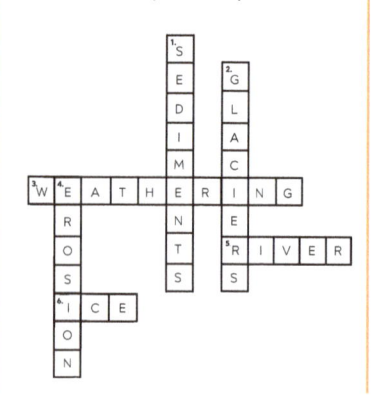

60 ANSWER KEY

Index of Skills

birthstones **34-35, 36**

crystals **25, 26, 27, 28, 29, 30**

Earth's layers **4-5, 6**

earthquakes **4, 40-41, 42**

erosion **55, 56-57**

fluorescent **16-17, 18**

fossils **7, 8, 37, 38-39**

gems **31, 32-33, 34-35**

geodes **28-29**

igneous rocks **7, 8, 10-11, 12**

lava **7, 10, 43, 44**

magma **4, 7, 10-11, 43, 44, 48**

metamorphic rocks **7, 8, 10-11, 12**

minerals **13, 14-15, 16-17, 18-19, 20, 22-23, 24-25, 28, 31**

mountains **46-47, 52, 54, 57**

rivers **49, 50-51**

rocks **7, 8-9, 10-11, 12-13, 19, 20, 22, 24-25, 28-29, 30-31, 37, 46, 52, 54-55, 56**

rock cycle **10-11, 12**

sedimentary rocks **7, 8-9, 10-11, 12**

tectonic plates **40-41, 46, 48**

volcanoes **10, 43, 44-45**

weathering **52-53, 54-55, 56-57**

61

About the Author

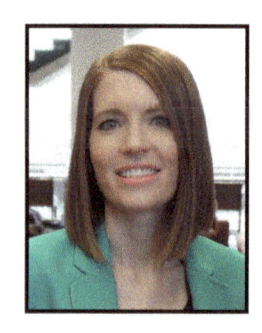

MEGHAN VESTAL is the founder of the curriculum development company Vestal's 21st Century Classroom LLC and a former teacher. She has created hands-on curricula for thousands of teachers and schools around the world and designed unique professional development opportunities for teachers. Her educational programs have been recognized by the US Congress. She is also the author of *Geology for Kids: A Junior Scientist's Guide to Rocks, Minerals, and the Earth Beneath Our Feet* and *Bold Women in History: 15 Women's Rights Activists You Should Know*.

You can learn more about Meghan by visiting Vestal's 21st Century Classroom's website or YouTube channel.

CPSIA information can be obtained
at www.ICGtesting.com
Printed in the USA
JSHW010215140222
22844JS00001B/2

9 781638 780724